# What people are saying about
## BEAT Crohn's:

"This book will help patients, families, and healthcare practitioners as a practical resource and should enthuse them about the importance of nutrition in Crohn's disease and its relevance to children, young people, and adults. It will encourage practitioners to offer, and patients to expect to have offered, enteral nutrition as a primary therapeutic option, and as continued nutritional support when other treatments are required."

**R. M. Beattie, FRCPCH MRCP, Consultant Paediatric Gastroenterologist, Honorary Senior Lecturer in Nutrition, Southampton General Hospital, England, UK**

"This easy-to-read book comprises a comprehensive and balanced assessment of the role that enteral nutrition plays in the management of Crohn's disease in children and adults. Enteral nutrition has been a forgotten and neglected treatment for Crohn's disease in many parts of the world—this book should help to change this, and will help many people (patients and health professionals alike) to understand a little more about this therapeutic option."

**Associate Professor Andrew S Day, Paediatric Gastroenterologist, Sydney Children's Hospital and University of New South Wales, Sydney, Australia**

"I think this is the most detailed, accurate, best researched, most objective and beautifully written account of this topic I have come across......by quite a long way! It is a huge amount of work, laid out in a clear and accessible way and is a really informative text for both patients and healthcare staff. I myself would love a copy of this as a reference text for teaching and staff training."

**Dr. Robert Heuschkel, MBBS, MRCPCH, Consultant Paediatric Gastroenterologist, Addenbrookes Hospital, Cambridge, UK**

"Easy to understand for a lay reader and particularly a Crohn's disease patient. I really do think this book will be valuable to patients and their families."

Professor Colm Ó'Moráin, D.Sc., M.Sc., M.D., M.A., Dip. Imm.,
F.A.C.G., F.E.B.G., F.R.C.P., F.R.C.P.I., F.T.C.D.,
Consultant Gastroenterologist,
The Adelaide and Meath Hospital, Dublin,
Professor of Medicine, Dean of Health Sciences,
Trinity College Dublin

"The book is designed for the patient and family with Crohn's disease and provides not only a detailed role of the use of enteral nutrition in this disease but also a summary of other therapies. The information given is evidenced-based and balanced in the claims for the role of enteral nutrition. The author avoids the use of medical jargon or explains the jargon where appropriate. There are illustrative case histories to which patients can relate. I would certainly recommend it to all patients with Crohn's disease and colitis. Patients with irritable bowel syndrome who are wondering about nutritional therapy will also get information."

Khursheed N. Jeejeebhoy, F.R.C.P. (C), Ph.D.,
Staff Gastroenterologist, Division of Gastroenterology,
St. Michael's Hospital, Toronto,
Professor of Medicine, Nutritional Sciences and Physiology,
University of Toronto

# BEAT
# Crohn's!

# BEAT
## Crohn's!

### Getting to Remission
### with Enteral Nutrition

Discover the clinically tested non-drug treatment
for children and adults with IBD

*Margaret A. Oppenheimer*

**Solutions**
Long Island City, NY

Cover design by Peri Poloni-Gabriel, Knockout Design
(www.knockoutbooks.com).
Cover illustrations by Phil Scheuer, Phil Scheuer Illustration
(http://philscheuer.com).
Book interior designed by Beverly Butterfield, Girl of the West Productions
(www.girlofthewest.com).

**Publisher's Cataloging In Publication**
Oppenheimer, Margaret A.
    Beat Crohn's! Getting to remission with enteral nutrition / Margaret A.
    Oppenheimer.—1st ed.
p.    cm.
    Includes bibliographical references and index.
    ISBN-13: 978-0-9821234-4-7
    ISBN-10: 0-9821234-4-2
    LCNN: 2009900983
    1. Crohn's disease.  2. Diet therapy.  3. Inflammatory bowel diseases.
    I. Title

RC862.E52 O67    2009
616.3'445—dc21

*To all those who strive to live well*
*with chronic disease*

# CONTENTS

# A NOTE TO
# HEALTH-CARE PROVIDERS

❖

This book was written for the general reader. It presents enteral nutrition in a positive light, but attempts to be honest about its limitations. Given its primary audience, it does not include probability figures, confidence intervals, or similar scholarly appurtenances. However, throughout the book any result referred to as significant meets conventional standards of statistical significance ($P < 0.05$). Remission rates were calculated based on intent-to-treat populations, whenever they could be ascertained.

All references cited in short form in the endnotes may be found in the bibliography. The bibliography also includes selected additional references consulted during the preparation of this book that may interest those curious about enteral nutrition. As the scope of the bibliography testifies, enteral nutrition is by no means an untested therapy, in spite of the modest size of many of the studies that explore it. I hope this book will spur further research into a treatment that is sometimes overlooked.

## ❖ 1 ❖

# What is
# Enteral Nutrition?

*Rebellions of the belly are the worst.*
**Frances Bacon**

This book describes a treatment for Crohn's disease that involves using **enteral nutrition**—special liquid formulas—to get into remission, stay in remission, gain weight, and reverse nutritional deficiencies.

Enteral nutrition has been prescribed by doctors for patients with Crohn's disease since the late 1960s, and has been evaluated in numerous clinical trials from the 1980s through the present. It has been tested in kids and adults, in patients with both recent and long-standing disease, and in individuals with many different complications of **inflammatory bowel disease** (**IBD**). Like all treatments for Crohn's, it doesn't work for everyone. But when it does, here are some of the things it can do:

- Enteral nutrition can induce remission in people with active Crohn's disease in as little as two weeks.
- Enteral nutrition can succeed in people who don't respond to steroids and those who can't discontinue steroids without relapsing.
- Enteral nutrition can restore normal growth patterns in kids who have stopped growing because of Crohn's.

1

- Enteral nutrition can promote healing in diseased areas of the intestinal tract.
- Enteral nutrition can do these things with almost no side effects.

## So why haven't I heard about enteral nutrition?

Well, there is one disadvantage to enteral nutrition. If you want to use it to get into remission from Crohn's (as opposed to taking it simply to maintain remission or gain weight), you can't eat or drink anything except the liquid formula for approximately two to eight weeks. You won't starve—the formula fills you up and provides all of your nutritional needs—but you do have to be willing to give up your regular diet temporarily.

Gastroenterologists in United States rarely mention enteral nutrition as a treatment option because they think it is too difficult to ask patients to give up normal food for a while. You are more likely to have heard about enteral nutrition if you live in Canada, Europe, Japan, or Israel. Doctors in these regions tend to have more experience using enteral nutrition for Crohn's, and are more likely to be aware of its benefits.[1] The Japanese, for instance, use enteral nutrition as a primary therapy for active Crohn's disease and prefer it to steroids.[2] In the United Kingdom, a survey of the members of the British Society of Gastroenterology found that 59% of the specialists who responded had prescribed enteral nutrition for their patients with Crohn's.[3] But in most countries, enteral nutrition is not used as often as it might be. If doctors consider prescribing it at all, they tend to offer it primarily to children because of its beneficial effects on growth, and rarely mention it as a treatment possibility to their older patients.

In part, this useful option may be overlooked because it's just too simple in a modern medical world that focuses on the complex. It's not a hot new treatment; it's been around for a long time, and many of us—doctors included—tend to look for the newest high-tech solution. To be honest, it's also much easier for a patient to take a medication every day than to comply with a liquid diet. Doctors realize this, and want to prescribe the treatment that is easiest for the patient. There are a fair number of drugs available to treat Crohn's disease, and they can be very effective for many individuals. So why not use them?

The trouble is that the medications don't work for everyone, and even when they do, can have unpleasant side effects. They can also lose their beneficial effects over time. That means that patients with Crohn's disease need to know about *all* their treatment options, just in case the simplest and most convenient methods fail. Enteral nutrition isn't appealing to everyone and doesn't work for everyone. Nevertheless, it is important for patients to know that it exists. That's why I wrote this book.

## What will I learn?

- In this chapter, we will learn what enteral nutrition is, who developed enteral nutrition and why (hint: NASA was interested!), and explore some of the hypotheses on why it works.

- In Chapter 2, we will look at the pluses and minuses of the drugs most commonly used to treat Crohn's disease, and explore why and when you might want to consider using enteral nutrition instead.

- In Chapter 3, we will discover the benefits of enteral nutrition in children with Crohn's.

- In Chapter 4, we will explore the advantages of enteral nutrition for adults, including its use during pregnancy.

- In Chapter 5, we will review the use of enteral nutrition for specific complications of Crohn's disease, such as perianal disease, fistulas, and strictures.

- In Chapter 6, we will examine whether enteral nutrition is useful in ulcerative colitis, indeterminate colitis, irritable bowel syndrome (IBS), and celiac disease.

- In Chapter 7, we will learn about the different types of enteral nutrition, and find out how each of us can choose a formula that is right for us.

- In Chapter 8, we will get the scoop on how to get started and what to expect during a course of enteral nutrition.

- In Chapter 9, we will examine whether people with Crohn's can benefit from other dietary regimens and supplements such as fish oil, probiotics, and low- or high-fiber diets.

## Understanding enteral nutrition

"Enteral nutrition" is not a phrase that's in most people's vocabulary, so before looking at what enteral nutrition does and how it can help you, let's take the time to better understand what it is.

Broadly speaking, enteral nutrition refers to any form of food or beverage delivered directly to the gastrointestinal tract, whether it is chewed and swallowed like normal food, or delivered through a tube directly into the stomach or intestines. Believe it or not, if you ate a sandwich and an apple and a soft drink for lunch, you were consuming enteral nutrition!

But when the term "enteral nutrition" is used in a medical context, it has a more specific meaning. In that case, it refers to special liquid diets used to feed patients who are too sick to eat regular food, or who would benefit medically from replacing normal food with a liquid formula, even if they can eat without difficulty. The formulas are supplied either as powders ready to be mixed with water, or already premixed (in liquid form). They provide all the nutrients that you would otherwise obtain from a varied diet.

There are many different enteral nutrition formulas to choose from, but they are usually divided into three main categories—**elemental**, **semi-elemental**, and **polymeric**—based on the form of protein they provide.

- Elemental formulas contain amino acids, the most basic ("elemental") building blocks of protein.
- Semi-elemental formulas contain small peptides (amino acids linked together into short chains), or a mixture of small peptides and amino acids.
- Polymeric formulas contain whole protein (made up of long chains of peptides).

We'll learn more about the differences between the types of formulas in Chapter 7. But for now, all you need to remember is that elemental, semi-elemental, and polymeric formulas are all considered enteral nutrition, and they all work equally well in people with Crohn's.

## A (very) brief history of enteral nutrition

Special types of liquids have been used for centuries to feed people who are ill and can't manage normal food. If you were tending a bedridden child or parent a few hundred years ago, you might have given them wine or brandy, or milk or eggs, or broth made from chicken or grain.[4] By the nineteenth century, doctors had even figured out how to use rubber tubing to get liquids straight to the stomach or intestines.[5] But the trouble was that none of these liquids were nutritionally complete. They weren't suitable for long-term use for patients who couldn't eat any other food because they didn't provide all the protein, fat, carbohydrates, vitamins, and minerals that a person needs on a day-to-day basis to stay alive.

The first extended experiments with enteral nutrition formulas that could supply all the nutrients required for human life began in the 1950s. A series of studies performed at the U.S. National Institutes of Health (NIH) and published in 1957 showed that rats could grow, thrive, and reproduce when consuming nothing except amino acid-based elemental diets.[6] The first reports of tests in human patients were published in the 1960s.[7] A key question was whether enteral nutrition formulas could really totally replace all other food for extended periods of time. That question was answered affirmatively in 1964, thanks to prisoners at a California jail who volunteered for a study. Fifteen men received no food except an elemental diet for five months, yet maintained normal weight and nutritional status.[8]

Believe it or not, some of the early research into enteral nutrition was supported by the U.S. National Aeronautics and Space Administration (NASA).[9] With the goal of sending men into outer space for days at a time, NASA had to figure out how to feed its astronauts. After all, you couldn't just send them to the nearest supermarket to refuel. A food suitable for astronauts needed to have certain characteristics. It had to have a long shelf life and be compact to store. Ideally, it would also be low-residue—that is, mostly absorbed by the body so that little remains to be excreted—to minimize the problem of disposing of human feces in space. An elemental diet seemed to be a winner on all counts. A single cubic foot of the powdered formula, when dissolved in water, could feed a 154-pound astronaut for a month, providing a nutritionally complete, low-residue regimen of 2,830 calories per day.[10] Because of NASA's interest in elemental diets, early publications about enteral nutrition formulas sometimes refer to them as "space diets" or "aerospace diets" or even "astronauts' diets."[11]

From a medical standpoint, enteral nutrition formulas were developed to provide nutritional support to any hospitalized patients who couldn't eat solid food. But doctors soon realized that these products might be particularly useful for individuals with digestive conditions that interfered with normal food absorption.[12] Enteral nutrition formulas have been used in patients with Crohn's disease since at least 1969.[13]

The big surprise was that patients with Crohn's not only improved nutritionally on enteral nutrition, but sometimes even went into remission or no longer needed scheduled surgery after being on one of these liquid diets.[14] The unexpected findings prompted researchers to conduct randomized, controlled clinical trials to establish whether enteral nutrition was a valid treatment for Crohn's disease. Those trials, along with other clinical studies and case reports discussed in the following chapters of this book, revealed the following:

- **Total enteral nutrition** (that is, not eating any food except an enteral nutrition formula for given period of time) can be as effective as steroids such as prednisone or prednisolone in inducing remission in children with Crohn's.

- It may not be quite as effective as steroids in adults with Crohn's, but still induces remission in some 50% or more of adults who are willing to comply with the treatment.

- Patients who relapse whenever their dose of steroids is lowered or withdrawn may be able to discontinue steroids with the help of total enteral nutrition.

- Total enteral nutrition can induce remission in some people who do not respond to steroids.

Fortunately for those who don't want to give up regular food, even temporarily, the studies also show that:

- **Supplemental enteral nutrition** (using an enteral nutrition formula to supply a portion of one's daily calories while continuing to eat a normal diet) can help people with Crohn's disease stay in remission longer.

- It can help malnourished patients gain weight and reverse nutritional deficiencies.
- It can restart growth in children with delayed growth due to IBD.
- It can help some people discontinue steroids.

Does enteral nutrition cure Crohn's? No. Unfortunately, nothing does. Some people who have mild disease may be lucky enough to only have a few flares, and then remain in remission for many years. But that doesn't mean that the disease is gone; once someone has Crohn's, he or she has it for life. That's why it's considered a chronic disease.

Enteral nutrition is one way to manage this particular chronic condition. It is very useful in helping many people with Crohn's achieve remission. There is no guarantee that it will work for you. Like all the different drugs used to treat Crohn's disease, it is effective in some people and not in others. There are also no guarantees as to how long remission will last; that varies from person to person. Some people are lucky and have a one- or two-year remission after a course of total enteral nutrition. Others are unlucky and relapse in a month. But enteral nutrition can be used more than once. Many people who find it effective return to it when they relapse, and then go back to regular food once they are in remission. Others don't want to try total enteral nutrition, but use enteral nutrition supplements to help stay in remission, prevent weight loss, or for kids, improve growth.

## Is this the same thing as TPN?

If you have had Crohn's disease for a while, you may have heard of, or used, **total parenteral nutrition**, called **TPN** for short. Parenteral and enteral nutrition are both ways of feeding people, but they are not exactly the same thing.

- Parenteral nutrition is liquid food given intravenously—straight into the bloodstream—through a catheter (slender tube) inserted into a vein.

- Enteral nutrition is liquid food that is drunk by mouth or delivered by a tube directly to the stomach or the intestines.

Going on total parenteral nutrition, or TPN, means receiving only intravenous feeding and no regular food, just as using total enteral nutrition means consuming no food except an enteral nutrition formula.

Both TPN and total enteral nutrition can induce remission and reverse malnutrition in patients with Crohn's. However, doctors tend to prescribe TPN rather than total enteral nutrition for seriously ill patients. They assume that enteral nutrition is less effective or impossible to tolerate in patients who are reluctant to eat. Or they may consider it less sophisticated, less high-tech, and therefore less valuable.[15] But total enteral nutrition is just as effective as TPN in most people with Crohn's, including those who are ill enough to need hospitalization. Six different studies, including a total of 293 patients with Crohn's, compared TPN with enteral nutrition. Uniformly those studies found that total parenteral and total enteral nutrition (whether with elemental, semi-elemental, or polymeric formulas) were *equally effective* in producing remission.[16]

They're not equal when it comes to safety, however. In that realm, enteral nutrition is the big winner. With enteral feeding the food goes directly into the intestinal tract rather than into the blood. That allows you, the patient, to avoid the risk of dangerous complications like blood clots and septicemia (overwhelming infection) that are associated with intravenous feeding.[17] Additionally, long-term TPN use can harm the liver, while any liver function abnormalities that occur during enteral nutrition tend to be mild and transient.[18]

❖ As long as your intestines are functioning even in part, total enteral nutrition works just as well as TPN, without the safety worries of parenteral nutrition.[19]

That's why this book focuses on enteral feeding. But we'll talk more about the choice between TPN and enteral nutrition in Chapter 8, and look at the special situations in which you might need TPN.

# Why does enteral nutrition work?

The short answer: nobody knows. There have been numerous attempts to find out, but the answer is still not clear. For those who are curious, here are some of the theories.

## Beating the bacteria

One speculation is that enteral nutrition formulas work because they reduce the number of bacteria living in the intestinal tract. Or perhaps they change the balance of bacteria, favoring species that help the intestines stay healthy. In fact, an early study found a dramatic decrease in the number of bacteria in the feces of healthy folks given an elemental diet.[20] Yet later studies found just the opposite: total enteral nutrition had little effect on the number and types of bacteria in stool.[21]

Nevertheless, the intestinal bacteria hypothesis hasn't been abandoned completely. A recent investigation found that the range of bacterial species in feces changed considerably as children treated with total enteral nutrition passed from active disease to remission. In contrast, an untreated control group of healthy children had stable patterns of fecal bacteria.[22] However, this small study is far from the last word in the matter. Is total enteral nutrition effective *because* it alters the bacterial balance, or do fecal bacterial patterns change as a side effect of going into remission, regardless of the way in which remission is achieved? We don't know.

## Giving the gut a rest

Another theory is that giving the intestinal tract a chance to rest and heal might be one of the keys to the success of enteral nutrition. Since most of the formulas typically used in people with Crohn's are fiber-free, the colon doesn't have to ferment as much food residue and the amount of stool produced is greatly reduced.[23] But if it's resting the gut that makes the difference, why isn't TPN more effective than total enteral nutrition? After all, delivering food straight to the bloodstream bypasses the intestinal tract far more completely than a liquid diet.

## Keeping out foreign proteins

Another potential explanation rests on the theory that some of the damage caused by Crohn's could be due to proteins from food passing through the ulcerated intestinal wall and setting off an inflammatory immunological reaction, with the body producing antibodies to defend against the "foreign" invaders (i.e., the many different types of protein in our diet). Perhaps elemental diets work because they only contain amino acids, and the body isn't exposed to all of those foreign proteins?[24] Or perhaps not. It turns out that people with Crohn's improve on enteral nutrition formulas that contain peptides or even whole protein. Semi-elemental and polymeric formulas work just as well as the amino-acid-based elementals.[25] Reducing the load of whole protein delivered to the gut might not be so important after all.

But this hypothesis hasn't been discarded entirely. When you consume an enteral nutrition formula as your only food for days at a time, your digestive tract is exposed to vastly fewer types of protein than when you are eating a normal varied diet, even if you are using a polymeric (whole protein) formula.[26] It's possible that the reduction in exposure to food proteins plays a part in the efficacy of enteral nutrition.

## Reversing malnutrition

It is equally plausible that the beneficial effect of enteral nutrition is due largely to the nutritional support that it provides. There is no question that enteral nutrition formulas are exceedingly effective in reversing the weight loss and nutritional deficiencies that are so common in those with Crohn's. Just getting back to a healthy weight can make a big difference in managing gastrointestinal diseases. Even in people without autoimmune diseases like IBD, malnutrition can affect the way in which the immune system functions, causing impairments that can be reversed by restoring normal nutritional status.[27]

Yet there are problems with attributing all the benefits of enteral formulas to the nutritional supplementation that they offer. Consider these two intriguing findings:

- The average growth rate in children who received intermittent treatment with total enteral nutrition increased from 1" to 3⅔" per year, even though they didn't consume any more calories during the year of intermittent enteral nutrition than during an observation year that preceded it.[28]
- Total enteral nutrition can reduce disease activity and inflammation in patients who begin treatment with *normal* nutritional status, implying that better nutrition is not the decisive factor in their improvement.[29]

Furthermore, if enteral nutrition works primarily because it reverses malnutrition, then why isn't a normal nutrient-rich diet as effective as enteral nutrition in jumpstarting growth and inducing remission?

## Reducing inflammation

The answer seems to be that enteral nutrition has an anti-inflammatory effect, although *how* it exerts that effect is unknown. The effect on inflammation was demonstrated clearly in a study of children with active Crohn's disease who were treated with total enteral nutrition. Within three days of starting treatment, the children showed a significant decrease (improvement) in **erythrocyte sedimentation rate (ESR)**, a blood test commonly used to measure inflammation in patients with Crohn's disease. Within seven days of starting the formula, **C-reactive protein**, another marker of inflammation, had decreased significantly, too.

In contrast, measures of nutritional status did not begin to improve significantly until the children had received enteral nutrition for two weeks or more.[30] In short, inflammation decreased *first*, and nutritional improvement *followed*, perhaps made possible by the reduction in inflammation.

A study in adults also found that most patients experienced decreased inflammation before any nutritional changes were apparent.[31]

There are other signals that total enteral nutrition is effective in reducing inflammation.

- Total enteral nutrition can reduce the production of cytokines (small proteins produced by cells of the immune system) that cause inflammation, such as tumor necrosis factor-$\alpha$ and interleukin-1$\beta$.[32]

- It can normalize levels of another protein, orosomucoid, that may be elevated when inflammation or tissue damage is present.[33]

- Endoscopies and x-rays performed before and after enteral nutrition treatment have shown improvement, and in some cases even complete healing, of diseased areas of the intestines. Biopsies have shown improvement on a microscopic level.[34]

- Scintigraphic scans, which track the movement of white blood cells to inflamed areas, have shown marked improvement in small and large intestinal inflammation in patients who responded to treatment with total enteral nutrition.[35]

The reduction in inflammation is probably responsible for a number of other changes that take place when total enteral nutrition is used. For instance:

- Total enteral nutrition can reverse, often completely, abnormal intestinal permeability that frequently accompanies active Crohn's disease.[36]

- Total enteral nutrition can reverse severe protein loss that often occurs during a flare of Crohn's.[37] It reduces the breakdown of protein on the one hand and increases the synthesis of new protein on the other.[38]

- Total enteral nutrition can speed up, and in some cases even completely normalize, intestinal transit time (which can be far slower in patients with active Crohn's disease than in healthy people).[39]

- Total enteral nutrition can improve the reabsorption of bile acid (important to the digestion of fats), reducing bile acid-induced diarrhea.[40]

- Total enteral nutrition can increase the production of insulin-like growth factor, a protein that stimulates growth, in children with Crohn's.[41]

Although it's likely that all of these benefits are secondary to the anti-inflammatory effect of enteral nutrition, we are still left with the basic question, why are these formulas anti-inflammatory at all? Possibly changes in the foods passing through the gut or the effects of those foods on the bacterial content of the intestines can affect the way in which genes are expressed in the outermost layer of tissue (**epithelium**) that lines the intestines. In turn, these changes could affect the way in which the immune system functions in the epithelium.[42] But this is only speculation. We've been using enteral nutrition in Crohn's disease for 40 years, and we still don't know exactly why it works! Still, what matters most is that it does work. In the following chapters we'll look at the studies that prove it.

## WHAT HAVE WE LEARNED?

❖ The term "enteral nutrition" is used to describe special liquid diets used for medical reasons instead of, or in addition to, regular food. Enteral nutrition formulas are categorized into three main types—elemental, semi-elemental, and polymeric—based on the form of protein they contain. All three types work equally well for people with Crohn's.

❖ Using total enteral nutrition involves eating and drinking nothing except an enteral nutrition formula for a certain period of time. Total enteral nutrition can induce remission in people with Crohn's, heal intestinal inflammation and ulcerations, and offer an alternative to steroids.

❖ Using supplemental enteral nutrition involves getting a portion of one's daily calories from an enteral nutrition formula while continuing to eat a normal diet. Supplemental enteral nutrition is an effective maintenance therapy for Crohn's, improves growth in kids with Crohn's, and is a good way to gain weight and reverse nutritional deficiencies.

❖ Enteral nutrition has an anti-inflammatory effect in the gastro-intestinal tract and can reverse abnormal intestinal permeability. It reduces protein breakdown and increases the synthesis of new protein, and can normalize intestinal transit time in people with Crohn's.

Most of the remaining chapters of this book explore enteral nutrition in more detail. But first, in Chapter 2, we'll take a look at the other treatments available for Crohn's and assess why and when you might choose enteral nutrition instead.

# ❖ 2 ❖

# Checking Out
# the Competition

## Treatment Options for Crohn's

*He who has health, has hope, and he
who has hope, has everything.*
**Thomas Carlyle**

Enteral nutrition is one way to treat Crohn's disease, but it is by no means the only option. This chapter offers an overview of other commonly used therapies for Crohn's. We'll explore:

- aminosalicylates for mild or moderate disease
- corticosteroids for attacking acute flares
- antibiotics for treating perianal disease and fistulas
- immunomodulating drugs for long-term disease control
- biologic drugs for treating severe or resistant disease
- the option of surgery when medications fail.

We will consider each treatment's approximate likelihood of inducing remission. We'll also weigh whether it is effective as a **maintenance therapy** (a treatment used on a long-term basis to maintain remission) and whether it can heal perianal disease and fistulas (common complications of Crohn's). In addition, we will briefly review the potential side effects of each therapy.

At the end of the chapter, we'll explore the place of enteral nutrition among these treatment options, and consider why and when you might prefer it to medication or surgery.

# Aminosalicylates

**Aminosalicylates** (ah-MEAN-oh-suh-LIS-ih-lates) are mild drugs that are often the first treatment prescribed to people with Crohn's. They are called aminosalicylates, or **5-ASA drugs** for short, because they contain an anti-inflammatory substance known as 5-aminosalicylic acid.

The first aminosalicylate tested in Crohn's disease was **sulfasalazine** (Azulfidine). Sulfasalazine is a medication that combines 5-aminosalicylic acid with an antibiotic, sulfapyridine.

Because some people are allergic to sulfapyridine, other aminosalicylates were developed that contain 5-aminosalicylic acid without the sulfapyridine. These drugs include:

- mesalamine (Asacol; Pentasa; Lialda; Rowasa; Canasa)
- olsalazine (Dipentum)
- balsalazide (Colazal).

## Sulfasalazine

**Sulfasalazine** (sull-fuh-SAL-uh-zeen) has been used to treat Crohn's disease for decades. It's sold under a number of different brand names in the US, including Azulfidine, Azulfidine EN-tabs, and Sulfazine EC, and in Canada as Alti-Sulfasalazine, Salazopyrin En-Tabs, and Salazopyrin, among others.

Sulfasalazine can help people with Crohn's reach remission. In one study, 38% of patients who took sulfasalazine reached remission by the end of 17 weeks, compared with only 26% of those treated with a **placebo** (a treatment identical in appearance but without

---

### Why does one drug have different names?

Every drug has a **generic name**. The generic name (typically not capitalized) is the drug's official name. Once a drug is assigned a generic name, that name doesn't change. But besides a generic name, most drugs have one or more **brand names** (also called trade names or proprietary names). The brand name, often easier to pronounce and remember than the generic name, is the name the company will use to market the drug.

After a manufacturer's patent protection for a drug expires, other companies can apply for regulatory approval to market the product. If approval is granted, they can sell the drug under its generic name or under a new brand name they create. Ultimately the drug may be available from a number of different companies, some marketing it under its generic name and others using various brand names.

In this book, drugs that have been available for a long time and may have several brand names are referred to by their generic names. Newer drugs that have a single, well-known brand name are referred to by the brand name because that is the name most familiar to patients.

---

any therapeutic effect).[43] Sulfasalazine was also significantly more effective than a placebo in a study with six months of follow-up.[44]

We don't know for sure whether sulfasalazine helps to maintain remission if it is continued on a long-term basis. At least one study found that maintenance therapy with sulfasalazine reduced the likelihood that Crohn's would recur during the first two years after surgery, but several other studies found that it didn't prevent patients in remission from relapsing over one or two years.[45]

Because sulfasalazine appears to be primarily effective in patients with large intestinal involvement, it is a better choice if you have Crohn's in the large intestine or in both the small and large intestines than if you have small intestinal disease only.[46]

The most common side effects of sulfasalazine include headaches, nausea, vomiting, loss of appetite, gastric discomfort, and reversible infertility in men (due to sperm abnormalities that go away when the drug is stopped). Allergic reactions can occur in people who are allergic to sulfa drugs. Rarer potential side effects include fever, rashes, hives, pancreatitis, decrease in production of blood cells, and effects on the liver, kidneys, nervous system, or lungs.

## Other 5-ASA drugs

Besides sulfasalazine, the 5-ASA drug used most commonly in Crohn's disease is **mesalamine** (meh-SAL-uh-meen). (It's also called **mesalazine**, especially in Europe). Mesalamine is available in different formulations that are designed to delay the release of mesalamine from its outer coating until it reaches specific parts of the intestines.

- Asacol releases mesalamine in the **terminal ileum** (the very end of the small intestine) and the **colon** (the main portion of the large intestine).
- Pentasa releases mesalamine throughout the gastrointestinal tract.

In the largest published studies of mesalamine in people with an active flare of Crohn's disease, from 36% to 45% of the participants were in remission after 8 to 16 weeks.[47] In one large study, mesalamine (Pentasa) was significantly more effective than a placebo at inducing remission, but in another study of similar design it was not.[48]

It is not clear whether mesalamine is useful as a long-term maintenance therapy in Crohn's. Some studies that tested whether mesalamine was useful in maintaining remission found that it wasn't any more effective than a placebo, while other studies found it beneficial.[49] If mesalamine is useful in maintaining remission in Crohn's disease, the benefit is likely to be small.

Side effects reported by people using mesalamine are usually mild. They include headache, flatulence, abdominal pain, diarrhea, nausea, vomiting, and rash. More rarely, side effects can include cardiac hypersensitivity reactions (myocarditis and pericarditis), renal impairment, pancreatitis, and liver problems. Some people may be intolerant of mesalamine, and develop an acute reaction including cramps, abdominal pain, and bloody diarrhea, and occasionally other symptoms such as fever, headache, fatigue, itching, rash, and conjunctivitis.

Besides Asacol and Pentasa, which are taken orally, mesalamine is also available in the form of enemas (Rowasa) and suppositories (Canasa). These products are used to treat inflammation in the colon, but chiefly for people with ulcerative colitis rather than Crohn's.

Lialda, a new delayed-release, oral version of mesalamine, was also developed primarily to treat ulcerative colitis. So far, there are no published studies testing Lialda in people with Crohn's.

Other 5-ASA drugs taken orally—Dipentum (olsalazine) and Colazal (balsalazide)—target the colon only. Like mesalamine enemas and suppositories, they are mainly used for patients with ulcerative colitis. Dipentum was not any better than a placebo at preventing relapse in patients with Crohn's disease located in the colon or colon and ileum. The drug also caused more side effects than the placebo.[50]

## Corticosteroids

**Corticosteroids**, also called **glucocorticoids**, or **steroids** for short, have been mainstays in the treatment of Crohn's disease for decades. They decrease swelling and inflammation, and also reduce the activity of the immune system, which can be overactive in people with Crohn's.

Many different steroids are available. Those used most commonly in Crohn's disease are **prednisone, prednisolone,** and **methyl-prednisolone.** Some other steroids include hydrocortisone, cortisone, dexamethasone, betamethasone, and triamcinolone.

These drugs are sold under many different brand names. They are typically taken orally (as tablets or capsules), but occasionally are given **intravenously** (injected into a vein) in seriously ill patients.

Corticosteroids help people with Crohn's feel better fast. If you have a flare and you start on a course of steroids, you may notice improvement within as little as a day or two. After only four weeks of treatment, as many as 85% to 90% of patients may reach remission.[51]

---

### What's the difference between corticosteroids and anabolic steroids?

The corticosteroids used for medical purposes in Crohn's disease are not the same as the anabolic steroids that may be abused by athletes or weightlifters. **Anabolic steroids** are synthetic versions of androgens, male sex hormones such as testosterone that are produced in the adrenal gland. Testosterone and other androgens make muscles large and strong, and stimulate the development of male sexual characteristics.

**Corticosteroids** are synthetic versions of a hormone called cortisol. Cortisol, like androgens, is produced in the adrenal gland, but has different functions. It regulates glucose levels and is released to combat stress. Corticosteroids do not improve athletic performance. They break down muscle and protein instead. In spite of that disadvantage, they are useful in IBD because of their anti-inflammatory effects.

In two longer studies, between 47% and 83% of patients taking steroids were in remission after four months, compared with only 26% to 38% of patients who received a placebo.[52]

As helpful as steroids can be in the short term, they are not recommended for long-term use. Over time, most people taking steroids tend to lose their response to the medication and relapse. Others become **steroid-dependent**, meaning that their disease remains under control as long as they continue treatment, but they relapse as soon as they stop taking steroids.

In one study of steroid-treated patients, 36% of those who initially reached remission became dependent on the medication within one year. An additional 20% no longer responded to steroids at all.[53]

In another trial, approximately one year after starting steroids only about a third of the patients had achieved prolonged complete or partial remission. A further 28% were dependent on steroids, and 38% had had to have surgery.[54]

❖ **Corticosteroids are no more effective than a placebo at maintaining remission over periods ranging from six months to three years.**[55]

## Side effects of corticosteroids

It's especially important not to be on steroids any longer than necessary because they can have unpleasant side effects, even with relatively short-term use. People taking steroids may bruise easily and develop stretch marks or acne. Having a ravenous appetite is common—a good thing in the short run if you've lost a lot of weight from Crohn's. But if you begin therapy at near your normal weight, you may find it difficult not to become overweight. Even those who do not put on the pounds may develop fat deposits on their upper back or a very round face (a complication graphically referred to as a "moon face").

Hair may grow on the face or back, even in women and young children. Insomnia and mood swings are common; people taking steroids may be nervous, restless, and quick to anger. Other possible complications of steroid use include muscle weakness, bone pain, water retention, diabetes, easy bruising, hypertension, slow wound healing, cataracts, glaucoma, and decreased resistance to infections. Long-term steroid use can lead to bone loss, even in young people.[56] Steroids may also suppress growth in children.

Because of this gamut of unpleasant side effects, most doctors try to avoid prescribing steroids for their patients except for short time periods, to treat an acute flare. But steroids are likely to remain an essential weapon in the treatment of Crohn's for the foreseeable future because of their powerful ability to control severe inflammation.

---

### A caution for those using steroids

If you are taking a course of steroids for Crohn's disease, *never stop treatment abruptly.* Your body monitors the total level of cortisol in the blood. It decreases its own cortisol production when you take steroids (a source of cortisol) for an extended period of time.

If you are ready to stop taking steroids, you need to reduce the dose slowly (a process known as tapering). That allows the adrenal gland time to begin producing normal levels of cortisol on its own again. Quitting steroids without gradually tapering the dose can be life-threatening.

---

## Budesonide—a different type of corticosteroid

The corticosteroids that we just discussed are considered **systemic steroids** because they affect the entire body (your whole "system," so to speak). An appealing alternative to systemic steroids is a controlled-release form of a corticosteroid called **budesonide** (byu-DES-in-ide) (Entocort EC; Budenofalk). First tested in Crohn's disease in the 1990s, budesonide in this controlled-release form is considered a nonsystemic steroid because it is active almost entirely in the intestines rather than throughout the body. Only limited quantities of the drug reach the bloodstream. Consequently steroid-related side effects are generally less frequent and less severe with budesonide than with systemic steroids such as prednisone or prednisolone—although the same range of side effects can still occur.

In patients with active Crohn's disease who used budesonide for eight to ten weeks, between 42% and 69% reached remission.[57] It was as effective as systemic steroids in six comparative trials.[58] But some people don't respond to budesonide and end up needing systemic steroids.

Like other steroid medications, budesonide is used primarily to treat acute flares of Crohn's, and is not suitable for long-term use. If you stay on it after reaching remission, it may help to maintain remission during the first three to six months of use, but it is no more effective than a placebo at warding off relapse by the end of a year.[59]

# Antibiotics

Antibiotics have been used for decades as a treatment for Crohn's disease, particularly for people with perianal disease and/or fistulas. Currently the two antibiotics used most frequently in Crohn's disease are **metronidazole** (meh-tro-NIDE-ah-zole) and **ciprofloxacin** (sip-roe-FLOX-ah-sin).

## Metronidazole

Metronidazole (Flagyl; Apo-Metronidazole) is the antibiotic that is best documented for use in Crohn's. In a four-month study, metronidazole was as effective as sulfasalazine at treating active Crohn's disease.[60]

---

**What are fistulas and perianal disease?**

**Fistulas** are passages that open up between areas of the body that would not normally be connected. For instance, a rectovaginal fistula may allow stool to pass from the rectum into the vagina. An enterovesical fistula may permit feces to pass from the intestines into the bladder.

**Perianal disease** refers to Crohn's symptoms affecting the anal and perineal area, such as fissures (tears in the skin) and ulcers. We'll talk more about fistulas and perianal disease in Chapter 5.

---

In two small series of patients, approximately 41% to 50% of fistulas closed during after three to 12 weeks of treatment with metronidazole.[61] In addition, evidence from **retrospective studies** suggests that as many as 72% to 91% of people using metronidazole achieve at least temporary improvements in perianal disease.[62] (See box below, **What is the difference between a prospective and a retrospective study?**)

Unfortunately, fistulas and perianal disease often recur once metronidazole is discontinued. Only 28% of the patients in one study could discontinue metronidazole without relapsing.[63]

The most common side effects of metronidazole are a metallic taste in the mouth and mild gastrointestinal symptoms (nausea, diarrhea, cramping, loss of appetite, vomiting). Drinking alcoholic beverages while taking metronidazole can cause more severe gastrointestinal symptoms and headaches and flushing. You should avoid drinking alcohol until at least one day after you have finished your course of treatment.

Metronidazole can cause peripheral neuropathy (nerve damage in the hands and feet), not always reversible, in as many as 50% of patients treated for six months or longer.[64] Rarer neurological side effects include seizures, dizziness, confusion, or depression. Because of the risk of neuropathy, metronidazole is generally used on a short-term basis only, but it remains one of the most effective treatments for Crohn's patients suffering from fistulas or perianal disease.

## Ciprofloxacin

Ciprofloxacin (Cipro; Cipro XR; Proquin XR) is another antibiotic used relatively frequently in Crohn's disease, although it is not as well studied as metronidazole. Limited evidence suggests that it can

---

### What is the difference between a prospective and a retrospective study?

**Prospective studies** enroll patients who have specific disease characteristics. They are giving a particular treatment at a predetermined dose, and observed to see what happens. The criteria used to determine whether someone has responded to the treatment are decided in advance.

Prospective studies may assess a single treatment, or they may compare two or more types of treatment. The most valuable evidence comes from randomized, double-blind, placebo-controlled studies—prospective studies in which patients are randomly assigned to a treatment or a placebo, and no one knows who received what until after the study ends.

**Retrospective studies** examine the records of people who have already been treated. The evidence they provide isn't as valuable as results from prospective studies. But retrospective studies can supply useful data when a disease or disease complication is not very common, making it difficult to recruit patients for a prospective study.

help to induce remission in mild to moderately active Crohn's disease, possibly as effectively as metronidazole.[65]

Ciprofloxacin is sometimes used in combination with metronidazole. However, in at least one retrospective study, using the two drugs together wasn't any more effective than using one or the other alone.[66]

The most common side effects of ciprofloxacin include nausea, diarrhea, abnormal liver function tests, vomiting, and rash. Some other possible side effects include hypersensitivity reactions, dizziness or lightheadedness, sensitivity to natural or artificial sunlight, peripheral neuropathies, joint or tendon problems, and central nervous system side effects such as agitation, seizures, confusion, and depression.

# Immunomodulators

In people with Crohn's disease, the immune system seems to be too aggressive. Instead of just protecting us from viruses or bacteria that might make us ill, it attacks our own body as well. Immunomodulating drugs, also referred to as immunosuppressives, are designed to reduce the activity of the immune system to more normal levels.

The three immunomodulating drugs used most commonly in Crohn's disease are **6-mercaptopurine** (Purinethol; Puri-Nethol), **azathioprine** (Imuran; Azasan), and **methotrexate**. (Technically, corticosteroids are immunomodulators, too, but they are placed in a class of their own rather than in the immunomodulator category since they have a different mechanism of action.)

All of the immunomodulators are slow-acting drugs. It can take as long as three to six months to see improvement after starting 6-mercaptopurine, azathioprine, or methotrexate. Generally speaking, a patient with an active flare of Crohn's will need a quick-acting therapy such as a steroid or enteral nutrition to help them feel better quickly. But an immunomodulator started at the same time can improve the likelihood of being able to discontinue steroids, and can help maintain remission once it is achieved.

Probably the biggest disadvantage of the immunomodulators is that they can make people who use them a little more susceptible to infections. There may also be a slightly increased risk of cancer with long-term use, but if so, the increase in risk is probably very small.

## 6-Mercaptopurine

The immunomodulating drug 6-mercaptopurine (six-mer-kap-toe-PURE-een), known as 6-MP for short, was developed in the early 1950s to treat leukemia in children. It is used at much lower doses to treat Crohn's.

6-MP can help induce remission in patients who are dependent on steroids or don't respond to them.[67] In a large series of patients treated with 6-MP, 66% were able to discontinue steroids.[68] In another study, 53% of patients treated with 6-MP were able to discontinue steroids, compared with only 13% of those given a placebo.[69]

6-MP is a useful maintenance medication. In children who had just achieved remission from their first attack of Crohn's, 9% given 6-MP as a maintenance therapy relapsed during an 18-month period, compared with 47% who were treated with a placebo.[70]

Among adults who were started on 6-MP or a placebo after an intestinal resection, 6-MP was significantly more effective than the placebo in preventing relapses over the next two years. 6-MP also reduced the risk of **endoscopic recurrence** (the reappearance of damage to the walls of the intestine, as assessed using an instrument called an **endoscope**).[71]

6-MP can improve perianal disease in some people, and can close around 31% to 40% of fistulas.[72]

Potential side effects of 6-MP include allergic reactions, infections, nausea, headache, fever, hair loss, pancreatitis, liver damage, rash, and bone marrow suppression (decrease in production of red blood cells, white blood cells, and/or platelets). There may also be a slightly increased risk of cancer with 6-MP use, although a couple of large studies didn't find any more cancers in IBD patients who had used 6-MP than in those who had not.[73]

## Azathioprine

Azathioprine (aze-uh-THIGH-oh-preen), first synthesized in 1957, is a slow-release formulation of 6-MP.[74] 6-MP is released when azathioprine is broken down in the liver.

Like 6-MP, azathioprine requires time to take effect. When used in a study of patients with active Crohn's, only 36% of the participants were in remission after 17 weeks, and azathioprine was not significantly more effective than a placebo.[75]

Although azathioprine was also not more effective than a placebo after one to two years of use in this trial, other studies have found that it can help maintain remission when used on a long-term basis. In patients who started taking azathioprine during a course of steroids and continued to use it as a maintenance therapy thereafter, 42% were still in remission at 15 months, compared with 7% of patients who received a placebo during and after steroid treatment.[76]

In patients who had been in remission on azathioprine for at least two years, 85% of those who continued treatment avoided relapse for an additional 12 months, compared with 47% of those who stopped taking the drug.[77] Similarly, a study of patients who had taken azathioprine for at least six months found that the probability of relapse after an additional year was 5% in those who continued to take the medication, compared with 41% in those who did not.[78]

Azathiaprine can be useful for people who are having difficulty stopping steroids. In 69 steroid-dependent patients started on azathiaprine, 48 (70%) were in steroid-free remission after taking the drug for one year.[37] A small study showed considerable endoscopic improvement in the ileum and colon in patients treated with azathioprine for an average of two years.[80]

Azathioprine may be useful in controlling perianal disease.[81] In one study of patients with perianal disease, 68% of the participants had at least temporary improvement.[82] However, in a larger series of patients, perianal disease showed sustained improvement in only 29%.[83]

Potential side effects of azathioprine are similar to those seen with 6-MP. They include nausea, vomiting, diarrhea, fever, malaise, increased risk of infections, leukopenia (reduced number of white blood cells) and/or reduced platelet count, hair loss, rashes, pancreatitis, and liver damage. There may also be a small increased risk of cancer with long-term use of azathioprine.

## Methotrexate

Of the immunomodulators, methotrexate (meth-oh-TREX-ate) tends to be used less frequently in people with Crohn's than 6-MP or azathioprine, and there are fewer studies of its use in Crohn's disease. It is typically given as a once-a-week injection.

Methotrexate is also available in tablet form (TREXALL; Rheumatrex), but few studies have tested oral methotrexate in Crohn's. In two trials that tested 9 to 12 months of treatment with oral methotrexate in patients with steroid-dependent Crohn's, the medication didn't show a conclusive benefit over a placebo.[84]

There is clearer evidence that injectable methotrexate can induce remission in people with Crohn's. In patients not responding to steroids, 39% of those started on methotrexate were in remission and off steroids after 16 weeks, compared with 19% of those given a placebo.[85] In another study, 37% of patients with refractory Crohn's treated with methotrexate were in steroid-free remission after an average of 22 weeks.[86] In a group of steroid-dependent and steroid-resistant patients, 29% were able to discontinue steroids after using methotrexate for four months.[87]

Methotrexate can help to maintain remission, too. In patients who reached remission after four to six months of treatment with methotrexate, 65% of those who stayed on the drug were still in remission 40 weeks later, compared with 39% of those given a placebo.[88]

In a small group of patients with fistulas who had failed treatment with 6-MP or were intolerant to it, fistulas closed during methotrexate use in 25%.[89]

Although methotrexate is sometimes considered not quite as effective as 6-MP or azathioprine, it is difficult to make reliable comparisons. Almost all the studies of methotrexate enrolled people who had failed to respond to another immunomodulating drug or hadn't been able to tolerate it, so they may have been patients with more severe disease.

In a study that compared azathioprine and methotrexate directly, the two drugs seemed to be equally effective, although side effects were significantly more common with methotrexate.[90] In a trial comparing 6-MP with oral (rather than intravenous) methotrexate, the rate of noticeable side effects didn't differ significantly between the two drugs.[91]

Among the more common adverse reactions that have been reported in people using methotrexate (intravenous or oral) are mouth ulcers, nausea, vomiting, abdominal discomfort, malaise, leukopenia, low platelet levels, fever, and infections. Other possible side effects include rash, hair loss, dizziness, increased sun sensitivity, severe diarrhea, liver damage, methotrexate-induced lung disease, neurotoxicity, and severe skin reactions. There may be a small increased risk of lymphoma associated with methotrexate use. As with any injectable drug, methotrexate injections can cause complications including nerve injury, local irritation, buildup of scar tissue, and abscess formation.

Methotrexate should not be used by women during pregnancy or when planning to conceive. Men are generally advised to discontinue methotrexate ninety days before attempting conception.

# Biologics

The **biologics** are the newest class of drugs available to treat Crohn's disease. They are called biologics or biological drugs because they are made from living organisms or their products. Biologics currently available to US patients with Crohn's are infliximab (Remicade), adalimumab (Humira), natalimumab (Tysabri), and certolizumab pegol (Cimzia). All four of these drugs are genetically engineered in a process that begins with a single cell. They are designed to reduce the body's ability to produce inflammation by interfering with specific elements of the body's inflammatory response.

- **Remicade**, **Humira**, and **Cimzia** inhibit the production of **tumor necrosis factor-α (TNF-α)**, a protein made by the immune system that causes inflammation.
- **Tysabri** inhibits the activity of a protein called **alpha-4 integrin** that is also involved in the body's inflammatory process.

These biologic drugs can be very fast-acting. Some patients notice improvement after the very first dose. They are effective for initial induction of remission and as maintenance drugs to maintain remission. They can be used to control fistulas and perianal disease.

The biologics also have disadvantages. All are very expensive. They are less convenient than some of the other medications available for Crohn's because they cannot be taken as tablets or capsules, only by injection. Remicade and Tysabri are infused intravenously (into a vein) at a doctor's office, hospital, or specialized infusion center. Humira and Cimzia are injected subcutaneously (under the skin). Patients can administer Humira themselves at home. Injections of Cimzia are given by a health-care provider.

Because biologic drugs can become less effective after a patient has been taking them for a while, some people prefer to keep these medications in reserve and use them only if they are unable to achieve remission using other therapies.

The risk of serious side effects is a little higher with the biologic drugs than with the immunomodulators (6-MP, azathioprine, and methotrexate). Patients using biologic drugs have a slightly increased risk of some cancers and infections, including common infections like sinus infections and opportunistic infections (rare infections that do not usually affect people with healthy immune systems).

Some people who use a biologic drug build up antibodies to the medication. If this happens, the drug may have to be discontinued. As a way of preventing or slowing the production of antibodies, people taking biologics are often given an immunomodulating drug as well. The trade-off is that using two drugs that affect the immune system (or three if you are taking a steroid, too) may increase the risk of infections and other side effects compared with using one drug alone.

## Remicade

Remicade (rem-eh-CADE) was the first biologic drug to be approved for use in the US for the treatment of Crohn's disease. It is typically given as three initial infusions at 0, 2, and 6 weeks, followed by an infusion every 8 weeks.

After one to three doses of Remicade, 56% to 67% of patients reach remission.[92] In addition, among patients dependent on steroids, 67% to 75% are able to discontinue them after three doses of Remicade.[93] However, of those initially needing steroids who continue to take Remicade as a maintenance therapy, only 25% to 46% remain in steroid-free remission at the end of a year.[94]

Long-term therapy with Remicade can promote healing of damaged intestinal tissue in a substantial proportion of patients.[95] In one study, 50% of the patients had complete endoscopic healing (that is, no intestinal damage visible through an endoscope) after a year of regular Remicade use, compared with just 7% of those who received the medication only occasionally.[96]

Remicade can be particularly useful for people with fistulas. From 39% to 61% of fistulas are closed at 8 to 12 weeks, after three doses of Remicade.[97] Among patients who continue to take the drug as a maintenance therapy, from 38% to 46% of fistulas remain closed at the end of a year.[98]

Perianal disease can also respond well to Remicade, but tends to relapse if the drug is discontinued. In a study of patients who were in remission on Remicade for a year and then stopped treatment, only 34% of those with perianal disease remained in remission for a further 12 months, compared with 69% of those without perianal or fistulizing disease.[99] In another study, only 36% of people with perianal fistulas or ulcers who responded two or three infusions of Remicade were still in remission a year after the infusions.[100]

The most common side effects of Remicade are respiratory infections, rash, headache, coughing, and stomach pain. Rarer potential side effects include infusion-related reactions, serious infections, liver problems, decreased production of blood cells, new or worsening congestive heart failure, symptoms resembling those of lupus (a rheumatological disease), reactivation of hepatitis B virus in people who carry the virus, and neurological problems such as paresthesias (pins and needles sensations), weakness, vision changes, or seizures.

The risk of cancer is slightly increased. Additionally, a handful of cases of a rare and often fatal cancer called hepatosplenic T-cell lymphoma have occurred in children and young adults who were using Remicade together with 6-MP or azathioprine.

## Humira

Treatment with Humira (hue-MARE-uh) typically begins with two "loading doses" (that is, higher than usual doses)—a 160-mg injection followed by an 80-mg injection two weeks later—and then is given as a 40-mg injection every other week.

Among patients with moderate to severe Crohn's disease who no longer responded to Remicade or were intolerant of it, 21% reached remission after two doses of Humira, compared with 7% of patients who received a placebo.[101] Response was better in patients who had not received any prior TNF-α therapy, with 36% in remission after two doses of Humira, compared with 12% of patients treated with a placebo.[102]

Among those without prior TNF-α therapy who reached remission after two to four doses of Humira, continuing with maintenance treatment every two weeks extended the length of remission. After 56 weeks, 79% of those who received Humira maintenance therapy were still in remission, compared with 44% given a placebo.[103]

In another study, among patients who responded well to initial treatment with Humira but were not necessarily in full remission after the two doses, 36% who continued to receive the drug every other week were in remission after 56 weeks, compared with 12% treated with a placebo.[104]

Humira may offer modest benefit to people with fistulas. In a study of patients no longer responsive to or intolerant of Remicade, 23% of fistulas were closed at four weeks after two doses of Humira.[105] In contrast, two other trials found that two doses of Humira were no more effective than a placebo in closing fistulas.[106]

Longer treatment was somewhat more effective. In 64 patients with an initial response to Humira who had enterocutaneous or perianal fistulas, 30% of those who continued to take the medication every week or every other week had complete fistula closure, compared with 13% of those who received a placebo.[107]

The most common side effects in people taking Humira are infections such as sinusitis or upper respiratory infections, injection site reactions, headache, and rash. Other potential side effects include more serious infections, allergic reactions, lupus-like symptoms, exacerbation or new onset of demyelinating disease, reactivation of hepatitis B virus in hepatitis B carriers, exacerbation or new onset of heart failure, and a decrease in the production of red blood cells, white blood cells, and/or platelets. There is a small increase in cancer risk associated with use of Humira.

## Tysabri

Tysabri (tie-SAB-bree) became available in the US in 2008 for the treatment of Crohn's disease. Originally approved for the treatment of multiple sclerosis (MS), it was pulled from the market briefly after the occurrence of three cases of a rare and devastating brain infection, progressive multifocal leukoencephalopathy, in two patients with MS and one with Crohn's who were taking Tysabri along with other immunomodulating drugs. Since then, two additional cases have occurred in MS patients taking Tysabri without other immunomodulators.[108]

Because of the risk of this brain infection, the US Food and Drug Administration (FDA) limits the use of Tysabri for the treatment of Crohn's to people with moderate or severe disease who haven't adequately responded to, or haven't been able to tolerate, other standard treatments. Patients using the drug have to be enrolled in a special monitoring program, and generally should not take Tysabri at the same time as immunomodulating drugs such as 6-MP or azathioprine. They must be able discontinue steroids, if they are taking them, within six months of beginning treatment with Tysabri in order to continue using the biologic drug.

Given these restrictions, Tysabri is likely to be used less frequently to treat Crohn's than Remicade or Humira. The potential advantage of Tysabri is that it works differently in the body than Humira and Remicade—it inhibits alpha-4 integrin rather than TNF-α—so it may be a helpful treatment option for people who don't respond, or no longer respond, to drugs acting on TNF-α.

Tysabri is given as an intravenous infusion once every four weeks. In studies of Tysabri, between 26% and 37% of patients reached remission after receiving three infusions of the drug.[109]

A study of patients who were in remission 10 weeks after beginning treatment with Tysabri found that 44% of those who continued to receive the drug every four weeks were still in remission at week 36, compared with 26% of those in whom Tysabri was replaced by a placebo.[110]

The most common side effects of Tysabri include headache, fatigue, allergic reactions, bone and joint pain, urinary tract infections, respiratory tract infections, and rash. Other potential side effects include serious infections, liver damage, depression, diarrhea, stomach pain, and, as mentioned, progressive multifocal leukoencephalopathy.

## Cimzia

Cimzia (SIM-zee-uh) is the latest biologic drug to be approved in the US for the treatment of Crohn's. It is approved for use in adults who have moderately to severely active Crohn's and haven't responded adequately to conventional therapies. Treatment begins with three 400-mg doses of Cimzia given at 0, 2, and 4 weeks, followed by a 400-mg dose every 4 weeks in patients who responded to the initial series of injections.

In a 26-week study of Cimzia, 29% of patients given the drug were in remission at the end of the trial, compared with 18% of those given a placebo.[111] In another study, Cimzia was given as a maintenance therapy to those who responded well to an initial four weeks of treatment. Among those good responders, 48% who continued to receive the drug were in remission after 26 weeks, compared with 29% who were switched to a placebo.[112]

The most common side effects of Cimzia are upper respiratory infections, urinary tract infections, and joint pain. Other potential side effects include more serious infections, injection site reactions, allergic reactions, reactivation of the hepatitis B virus in people who carry it, exacerbation or new onset of neurological disorders, reduced production of red blood cells, white blood cells, and/or platelets, and development of a lupus-like syndrome. It is not yet clear whether there is an increased cancer risk associated with Cimzia use.

## Surgery

Surgery is used in patients with Crohn's whose symptoms cannot be controlled any longer with other treatments or who have life-threatening complications such as an intestinal blockage, perforation, or **abscess** (an infected, pus-filled area). Removing a diseased or obstructed portion of the intestine can induce remission, especially if the disease is localized to a single area. In addition, surgery can be very effective in restoring growth in kids with Crohn's. After a diseased section of bowel is removed, children frequently show dramatic gains in height and weight.

Unfortunately, surgery is not a permanent cure for Crohn's.

- Within a year of undergoing surgery, over 70% of patients have endoscopically detectable intestinal lesions.[113]
- Between 25% and 30% of surgically-treated patients will have another operation within five years.[114]

Other downsides of surgery are the risks, cost, and trauma involved, and the permanent loss of a section of intestine. People who have to have large amounts of intestine removed may have trouble absorbing nutrients, or may need a **stoma**, an artificial opening created in the abdomen for the excretion of wastes.

To minimize the risks of surgery, some less invasive techniques have been developed. Sometimes it is possible to widen rather than remove a narrowed section of intestine using a surgical procedure called a **stricturoplasty**. Alternately, a doctor may be able to stretch open a narrowed area with a special type of balloon. This procedure is called an **endoscopic balloon dilation**.

## How does enteral nutrition compare?

Now let's see how enteral nutrition stacks up. But since it is the focus of the remainder of this book, we'll stick to the highlights here. We'll look at total enteral nutrition and supplemental enteral nutrition separately, because these two ways of using enteral nutrition have their own advantages and disadvantages.

### Total enteral nutrition

Total enteral nutrition, as we learned in Chapter 1, is a dietary treatment for Crohn's disease. It involves eating or drinking nothing except a special liquid formula for a limited period of time—most commonly from two to eight weeks—in order to induce remission.

Total enteral nutrition is effective in treating acute flares of Crohn's. As with steroids, it can take effect quickly. Many people will start to notice improvement within the first few days of starting total enteral nutrition. The average time required to reach full remission ranges from 9 to 34 days.[115]

In the six largest prospective studies of total enteral nutrition, remission rates after two to eight weeks of treatment ranged from 41% to 77%.[116]

Total enteral nutrition can be effective in people who are **steroid-refractory** (don't respond to steroids) or **steroid-dependent** (can't discontinue steroids without relapsing). In small series of steroid-dependent patients, between 28% and 60% of patients who used total enteral nutrition were able to discontinue steroids.[117] Two small studies that included a mix of steroid-dependent and steroid-refractory patients found that up to 63% reached steroid-free remission on total enteral nutrition.[118]

Fistula closure is possible with enteral nutrition, but can require two months or more of treatment. In the largest published study of nutritional treatment of fistulas, 54 of 75 fistulas (72%) were completely closed after an average of 101 days of total enteral nutrition.[119]

Limited data suggest that perianal fissures and ulcerations can respond to total enteral nutrition. However, perianal fistulas can be quite difficult to close, and perianal disease may recur quickly after enteral nutrition is discontinued.[120]

At least partial healing of the **intestinal mucosa** (inner walls of the intestines) can occur in as many as 50% or more of patients who respond to a course of total enteral nutrition, with small numbers achieving complete healing.[121] Total enteral nutrition is significantly more effective than steroids at healing mucosal damage in the intestines.[122]

Side effects of total enteral nutrition are typically mild. Nausea, bloating, or mild abdominal pain may occur, mainly during the first few days after initiating treatment. Going for a long time without consuming any formula can cause headaches or dizziness.

Dehydration can cause constipation (easily reversed by drinking a little extra water). Diarrhea or nausea can result from drinking the formula too quickly or intolerance of a particular formula.

Severe side effects are rare. Refeeding syndrome, a potentially serious disturbance in the body's balance of fluids and electrolytes, can occur when people who are malnourished begin to receive proper nutrition. Also, a few cases of rhabdomyolysis (all reversible) have been reported in people using total enteral nutrition. Rhabdomyolysis causes muscle cells to break down and release a substance that can damage the kidneys. (See Chapter 8 for a more detailed discussion of the possible side effects of enteral nutrition).

The biggest disadvantage of total enteral nutrition is that it requires you to give up your normal diet temporarily. For most people, that's tougher than taking pills or an injection.

## Supplemental enteral nutrition

Supplemental enteral nutrition involves using an enteral nutrition formula to supply a portion of one's daily calories while continuing to eat a normal diet. Supplemental enteral nutrition can extend the length of remission. In two studies of Crohn's patients in remission, from 57% to 59% of people who supplemented their diet with enteral nutrition for a year remained in remission for the entire 12 months, compared with 21% to 22% of those who chose not to supplement.[123]

Supplemental enteral nutrition is generally not enough to achieve initial induction of remission. However, in one study of steroid-dependent patients, 42% were able to achieve steroid-free remission and maintain it for at least 12 months just by supplementing.[124]

For children and adolescents with delayed or slow growth due to Crohn's, supplemental enteral nutrition is highly effective at restoring normal growth patterns.[125]

There are few side effects to supplemental enteral nutrition. Some people experience mild nausea, bloating, abdominal pain, or diarrhea. As with total enteral nutrition, the main difficulty is with compliance. Some people dislike the taste of enteral nutrition supplements or object to having to take them on a regular basis.

## Why choose enteral nutrition?

There are many options for treating Crohn's disease. Most people with Crohn's will end up using a number of different treatments over time. Each is right at different times, in different people, and in different situations. No treatment for Crohn's disease works for everyone, every time.

There are a variety of reasons why you might choose enteral nutrition now or in the future. Here are 15 possibilities:

1. You like the idea of being able to control disease with nutrition rather than medications.

2. You've read about the side effects of the medications available to treat Crohn's, and you'd prefer to try a non-drug option first.

3. You're taking steroids and can't discontinue them without relapsing.

4. You'd like to postpone using biologics as long as possible because their benefits can decline with time. You want to save them until you really need them.

5. You've tried all the available medications for Crohn's, and nothing works for you any longer.

6. You would like to have a child, but you're worried about using Crohn's medications during pregnancy and breast-feeding.

7. You have persistently active disease and are unable to maintain your weight, no matter how much you eat.

8. You have limited ability to absorb nutrients because of prior surgeries for Crohn's.

9. You are being treated, or have been treated, for cancer, and you are worried that using immunomodulating drugs to treat Crohn's could increase your risk of a cancer recurrence.

10. You're worried about the risk of excessive weight gain from steroid use.

11. You have **osteoporosis** or **osteopenia** (weakened bones) and want to avoid medications that could cause further bone loss.

12. You suffer from depression or anxiety and want to avoid steroids because they could worsen your emotional state.

13. You have an acute flare of Crohn's, you're not responding to steroids, and your condition is too serious to wait for an immunomodulator to work. You want an alternative to starting a biologic drug.

14. You're looking for a safe long-term maintenance therapy for Crohn's.

15. Your child has stopped growing because of Crohn's and needs a treatment that will restore normal growth as well as control the symptoms of the disease.

## It's not a lifetime commitment!

Choosing to use enteral nutrition is not an irrevocable decision. Some people will try it once, find that it's not for them or doesn't work for them, and go on to use other treatments. Others will make it their first choice, using total enteral nutrition to treat flares and supplemental enteral nutrition as a maintenance therapy.

There is no right or wrong way to use enteral nutrition. Whether you use it, how often, and how much will depend on many factors:

- your level of comfort with dietary changes
- the amount of support you get from your doctor, family, and friends
- your personal feelings about the treatment that will best fit your lifestyle
- the range of therapies available to you at a given moment
- the degree to which your case of Crohn's responds to enteral nutrition.

## WHAT HAVE WE LEARNED?

❖ In this chapter, we learned about the various treatments for Crohn's disease. Options for mild disease include sulfasalazine and the other 5-ASA drugs. Corticosteroids, total enteral nutrition, and biologic drugs can be used to treat an acute flare.

❖ Maintenance treatments include immunomodulating drugs, biologics, and supplemental enteral nutrition. Possibilities for treating fistulas and perianal disease include metronidazole, immunomodulators, biologic drugs, and total enteral nutrition. Each treatment has its advantages and disadvantages and is appropriate in different situations.

❖ The biggest advantages of enteral nutrition are that it can be effective and quick-acting and has few serious side effects. The biggest disadvantage is that it requires changing your diet at least temporarily.

In the next two chapters we'll take a more detailed look at what enteral nutrition can do, focusing on children in Chapter 3 and adults in Chapter 4.

## ❖ 3 ❖

# Happy Kids,
# Healthy Bodies

## Enteral Nutrition for Children

*In children with Crohn's disease enteral nutrition is considered as the first-line therapy.*
**ESPEN Guidelines on Enteral Nutrition: Gastroenterology** [126]

Do you know a child with Crohn's disease? Then you need to know about enteral nutrition. As the treatment guideline above makes clear, enteral nutrition is an essential option for kids with Crohn's. Here are some of the things it can do:

- Enteral nutrition can get kids into remission.
- As a supplement to their normal diet, it can keep them in remission.
- It can help kids get off steroids without relapsing.
- It can promote healing of ulcerations and inflammation in the intestines.
- It has almost no side effects—none at all in many children.

Enteral nutrition also has a special benefit in youngsters. Growth slows down in many kids with Crohn's because of the inflammation caused by the disease. Enteral nutrition can get kids growing again, whether given as a replacement for a child's usual diet (**total enteral nutrition**) or as a supplement to normal food (**supplemental enteral nutrition**).

# A time-tested treatment

Enteral nutrition has been used safely for years. Promising reports of its use in kids with Crohn's began to appear in medical journals in the late 1970s and early '80s.[127] Doctors were struck by the fact that children who remained sick in spite of standard medications improved dramatically when total enteral nutrition was added to the mix.

For example, in 14 kids with Crohn's and poor growth, symptoms decreased in every child within one to two weeks of starting enteral nutrition. Blood tests showed reduced inflammation and better absorption of protein and iron.[128]

The children stayed on total enteral nutrition for a total of four weeks, and then gradually added back solid food over the course of six weeks while supplementing their diet with enteral nutrition. Some continued to use the formula afterwards as a nutritional supplement.

Within three months, three of the kids had grown substantially, and six had considerable increases in weight. Eleven of the 14 stayed in remission for between six months and three years.

Another intriguing report described a child with very severe Crohn's disease who failed to stay in remission using standard treatments (surgery, metronidazole, sulfasalazine, and steroids). During three months of total enteral nutrition, the child's symptoms disappeared, bloodwork normalized, and height and weight increased substantially. The youngster was still in remission two years later.[129]

# Comparing enteral nutrition and steroids

Once doctors realized that total enteral nutrition might help kids with Crohn's, it was time to perform controlled studies to find out just how effective it really was. That meant comparing enteral nutrition with steroids.

Why use steroids for comparison? After all, as we discussed in Chapter 2, steroids have some very unpleasant side effects: obesity, osteoporosis, insomnia, irritability, and others. But steroids are effective at treating flare-ups of Crohn's, even though they are not recommended for long-term use. When you test a new treatment, you want to compare it with something that works so you can see if the new therapy is better, worse, or equal to the old one.

Doctors compared enteral nutrition with steroids in children with Crohn's in six randomized studies. *All six trials found that the two treatments were equally effective in inducing remission.* The choice of formula didn't matter; two studies tested polymeric diets, three semi-elemental diets, and one an elemental formula.[130]

Total enteral nutrition was also as effective as steroids in inducing and maintaining remission in two retrospective studies (studies that looked at the records of children who were already treated, rather than randomly assigning them to the two therapies).[131]

> "Total enteral nutrition represents an effective alternative to corticosteroid therapy in the treatment of acute episodes of Crohn's disease, especially in the case of malnutrition."
> Nutrition Committee of the French Society of Pediatrics[132]

## How effective is enteral nutrition in children?

As many as 80% or more of children reach remission in some studies. Typically, however, enteral nutrition is not quite so effective across the entire population of kids with Crohn's. Some studies with high remission rates didn't include any children with **Crohn's colitis** (Crohn's disease limited to the large intestine), which appears to be somewhat less responsive to enteral nutrition than disease limited to the small intestine or mixed small and large intestinal disease.[133] (We'll take a more detailed look at which children are most likely to respond enteral nutrition later in this chapter.) Also, the studies with particularly high success rates were often small.[134] Patients enrolled in small studies may receive more encouragement to persist with treatment than those who participate in larger ones.

The two biggest prospective studies of enteral nutrition in kids had remission rates of 77% (among 65 children treated for eight weeks) and 57% (among 84 children treated for 20 days).[135] The larger study, with its 57% remission rate, probably best reflects the results you would achieve if you tested total enteral nutrition in a random selection of kids with Crohn's, with varying disease severity, disease location, and willingness to persist with enteral nutrition.[136] That said, a success rate of nearly 60%, achieved in spite of the fact that 10 kids dropped out because they weren't willing to comply with the treatment, is excellent in treating a difficult disease like Crohn's. And for those who do respond to enteral nutrition, improvement can be truly spectacular.

### Rob's Story

Ten-year-old Rob was diagnosed with Crohn's disease in his stomach and small intestine.[137] He had vomiting, fierce stomach pains, and fevers as high as 104°. He was immediately started on Pentasa (a 5-ASA drug), Entocort (a steroid), and an antacid. In spite of the treatment, he began to feel even worse. Within a month he was in constant pain, couldn't eat, and had such bad joint pain he couldn't walk. He had lost 14 pounds since his diagnosis and weighed only 51 pounds. His mother Irene said, "In my eyes, he was dying."

Irene searched for other treatments and learned about enteral nutrition. She obtained some samples of a formula, Modulen IBD. Rob tried to drink them, but he was so sick that he threw up whatever he managed to swallow. As an alternative, he was admitted to the hospital to have a nasogastric feeding tube inserted to make it easier for him to take the formula.

By the second day of enteral nutrition, Rob's pain was less severe and his temperature had returned to normal. His joint pain subsided over the next two weeks. By the end of three weeks of total enteral nutrition he was free of pain and had gained almost 3 pounds. Within another two and a half weeks all of his blood work was normal. By the end of two more weeks (after just over seven weeks of total enteral nutrition), Rob had gained back 11 of the 14 pounds that he had lost since his diagnosis, and was able to play basketball with his friends and ride his bike.

## Enteral nutrition restores normal growth

Many kids with Crohn's have growth delays, and some never reach their expected height (see box below, **The effects of IBD on growth**). Luckily enteral nutrition is highly effective at getting kids back on track with growth. *Every study comparing growth in children receiving total enteral nutrition or steroids has shown that the nutritional treatment produces significantly better gains in height.*[138] For instance:

- Among children treated with enteral nutrition for 12 to 15 weeks, growth soared from ⅓" per six months to almost 1½" per six months. The growth rate of a comparison group of children treated with steroids didn't change.[139]

- In another study, six of nine children who used total enteral nutrition experienced **catch-up growth** (meaning that they temporarily began growing faster than their healthy peers to made up for growth they had missed). Only one of eight children who took steroids had catch-up growth.[140]

The growth benefits of enteral nutrition can persist for months after a child returns to a regular diet. Among 10 children who were treated with total enteral nutrition for an average of three and a half months, eight grew during treatment, gaining an average of ¾" in height. They were still growing just as fast three months later. By nine months after treatment their growth rate had slowed, but it was still much greater than it had been before enteral nutrition.[141]

---

### The effects of IBD on growth

Before puberty, most children grow a minimum of 1 ½" (4 cm) per year. But kids with IBD, especially those with Crohn's, often grow a lot more slowly than their peers. They are also likely to start puberty significantly later.[142] As many as one-third of children with Crohn's disease may have periods when they do not grow at all for a year or more, a situation known as **growth failure**.[143] Even when they do eventually have a growth spurt, these children may never become as tall as their contemporaries.[144] A study that followed 48 children with IBD into adulthood found that 25% had final heights below 5'5" for the men and 5'1" for the women.[145]

Slowed growth may be the first sign of IBD. One study of children and teenagers with Crohn's found that 44 out of 50 had a decrease in rate of growth *before* they were diagnosed with Crohn's.[146] Being underweight is often part of the problem. Kids with Crohn's may be reluctant or unable to eat because of abdominal pain, diarrhea, or other gastrointestinal symptoms. But malabsorption due to the disease can cause nutritional deficiencies even in children eating an adequate diet.

In recent years, researchers have recognized that inflammation from the disease process itself can be a major factor in suppressing normal development. Inflammatory cytokines—

small proteins released by cells in the immune system—inhibit the production of insulin-like growth factor, a protein that stimulates growth.[147] Children usually begin growing again once the inflammatory process is stopped, whether by medications, enteral nutrition, or surgically removing a diseased portion of the intestines. But it's important to deal with growth problems promptly. Once a child has passed through puberty, it may be too late to make up for lost height.

Want to check how your child's growth compares with that of his or her peers? See the growth charts for boys and girls in Appendix A.

## Enteral nutrition can heal damaged intestinal tissues

Enteral nutrition can heal the ulcers that Crohn's disease causes in the **intestinal mucosa** (the inner walls of the intestines). Doctors assess this **endoscopically** (by looking at the appearance of the intestines through an instrument called an endoscope) and **histologically** (by taking samples of intestinal tissue—**biopsies**—and examining their appearance under a microscope).

- Among children who were randomly assigned to receive methylprednisolone or enteral nutrition for 10 weeks, there was significantly more mucosal healing with the nutritional treatment than with the steroid.[148]

- In another group of children treated for eight weeks with prednisolone, enteral nutrition, or cyclosporin A (an immunomodulating drug), biopsy-proven improvement of intestinal tissues was greatest after enteral nutrition.[149]

- In another study, endoscopic improvement in the ileum and colon was significantly greater after eight weeks of total enteral nutrition than after steroids, and significant histologic improvement occurred only with enteral nutrition.[150]

The degree of mucosal healing achieved after enteral nutrition varies. Small numbers of children achieve complete healing, larger numbers benefit from partial healing, and in others mucosal healing does not occur.[151] But even partial improvement is a considerable achievement. There is *little or no* endoscopic improvement of the intestines after steroid therapy.[152]

## Getting off steroids with enteral nutrition

What if your child is already taking steroids? If he or she has responded well and you are able to taper and discontinue the medication without provoking a relapse, steroids may turn out to be a good short-term treatment for your child. Some kids, however, become **steroid-dependent** (unable to discontinue steroids without flaring). This is a *big* problem, because steroids can cause major side effects if they are used on a long-term basis.

Luckily enteral nutrition can help children get off steroids without relapsing. In one study, 10 teenagers taking prednisolone were started on enteral nutrition. It was used as their only food during periods of disease relapse, and otherwise taken regularly as a supplement. Within four months, the prednisolone dose could be reduced in every child and six no longer required it. These six children were still in remission one year after starting enteral nutrition.[153]

Another study looked at 11 children and teenagers who had been referred for surgery for Crohn's disease, but chose to use total enteral nutrition as a way of postponing the operation to a more convenient time. They were treated for anywhere from five weeks to four and a half months. Although 10 of the 11 children were initially on prednisone (on average, 36 mg/day), 6 were able to discontinue it during enteral nutrition use and the remaining 4 were on significantly lower dosages (on average, only 6 mg/day). They all benefited from reduced symptoms, and four of the children ended up refusing the previously planned surgery.[154]

## How long will my child stay in remission?

There isn't any one answer to that question. Some children relapse within a week or two of resuming normal food. Others benefit from several years of remission after a single course of total enteral nutrition. Most fall somewhere between these extremes. For instance, among 10 children who received total enteral nutrition for approximately 3 ½ months, 7 achieved a remission lasting between 3 and 6 months, 1 stayed in remission for over 6 months, 1 for 15 months, and 1 for over 3 years.[155]

In another study, 34 children who responded to enteral nutrition when it was given as their initial treatment for Crohn's remained in remission for anywhere from 2.7 to 305 weeks, with the median duration being 21.4 weeks.[156] In another series of newly diagnosed children, remission lasted anywhere from 4 to 312 weeks.[157]

## How can I keep my child in remission longer?

It can be very disappointing to see a child relapse only a few weeks or months after completing a course of total enteral nutrition. That raises the question: Once your child has achieved remission, is there anything you can do to help him or her maintain it?

Staying on enteral nutrition long-term is one possibility. Several children who remained on total enteral nutrition for a year found that their intestinal symptoms disappeared and did not recur at any point during the year, even though they weren't taking any other treatment for Crohn's disease.[158]

Another patient, a teenager with delayed puberty due to Crohn's, was kept on total enteral nutrition on a long-term basis to help him grow and gain weight. At age 18 he weighed only 66 pounds and was just over five feet tall. Over the course of 54 weeks of nutritional treatment (three months of TPN followed by nine and a half months of total enteral nutrition and sulfasalazine), he gained 35 pounds, grew 2 ¾", began to produce normal levels of testosterone, and developed secondary sex characteristics.[159]

But many children will object (understandably!) to remaining on enteral nutrition on a long-term basis. A less demanding approach is to alternate regularly between total enteral nutrition and a normal diet. This technique is excellent at improving growth—significantly better than using steroids or various conventional treatments on their own.[160] Some evidence:

- Children who received total enteral nutrition for one of every four months for a year, along with conventional medical treatment, grew an average of 2 ¾". Those who received conventional medical treatment grew only ⅔" during the year.[161]

- Six children who used a similar schedule of total enteral nutrition every fourth month, alongside conventional medical treatment, increased their average growth rate from 1" to 3 ⅔" per year and their average weight gain from 6 ½ to 14 ½ pounds per year.[162]

In both these studies, the children using enteral nutrition also benefited from reduced disease activity and decreased need for prednisone.[163]

However, returning to total enteral nutrition on a regular cycle throughout the year, whether or not a child is experiencing a relapse, is a big commitment and may be unnecessary. After all, some children will remain in remission much longer than four months after a course of enteral nutrition. Yet the improved growth and reduced symptoms experienced by children using intermittent enteral nutrition is compelling. Luckily, there is an easier way to achieve those benefits. It's called supplemental enteral nutrition.

## Maintaining remission with supplemental enteral nutrition

**Supplemental enteral nutrition** means using enteral nutrition as a dietary supplement alongside regular food, rather than as a child's only food or beverage. Supplemental enteral nutrition can be just as effective at improving growth as total enteral nutrition, and may even prolong remission.

The best evidence for this comes from a hospital where children who achieved remission using total enteral nutrition were routinely instructed to resume an unrestricted normal diet, but encouraged to supplement it with enteral nutrition four to five nights a week. The supplements were given through a nasogastric tube, so the children could be fed while they slept. (See Chapter 8 for details about tube feeding.)

Records showed that 28 of 47 children and adolescents treated at the hospital agreed to use the supplements. For each nightly feeding, they used 50% to 60% of the amount of formula that they had consumed per 24 hours during the time when enteral nutrition was their only food.

After six months of supplementing, 23 of the 28 kids (82%) were still in remission. Sixteen (57%) were still in remission after an additional six months. In comparison, only four (21%) of the 19 children who didn't use the supplements were still in remission six months after completing their course of total enteral nutrition.

As an extra bonus, the participants who supplemented grew faster than before (2½" per year, compared with 1¼" per year before treatment). The growth rate of those who refused the supplements didn't change.[164]

# Supplemental enteral nutrition and growth

The children in the prior study began supplemental enteral nutrition after completing a course of total enteral nutrition. But supplements can be used on their own to improve growth, whether alone or in conjunction with conventional medications. That makes supplemental enteral nutrition a good choice if your child doesn't want to give up regular food, but does have growth delays or weight loss.

Usually those who are most consistent about using their chosen supplement are rewarded with the greatest improvements in height and weight.[40] The results can be dramatic. For example:

- A 14-year-old boy with Crohn's disease of the ileum and entire colon who had not reached puberty consumed enough enteral nutrition in addition to his normal diet to raise his total intake to 3,000 calories per day. *He gained 29 pounds in six months and grew 3 1/8" over 18 months of follow-up, after not growing at all in the year before treatment.*[165]
- An 11-year-old girl with steroid-dependent Crohn's disease involving the ileum and colon had not grown at all in a year. She received 500 calories a day of enteral nutrition for two months, and then 250 to 500 calories a day for six months. *She gained 11 pounds and grew 2 1/3".*[166]
- Five children supplemented their normal diet for 3 to 12 months with 600 to 1,200 calories a day of enteral nutrition. *They increased their average growth from 3/4" in the year before treatment to 2 1/2" during the treatment year.*[167]

## Can supplemental enteral nutrition induce remission?

Since supplemental enteral nutrition improves growth and helps to maintain remission, is total enteral nutrition necessary? Might children be able to reach remission by using a liquid diet for only part of their calorie intake, while still consuming a reasonable amount of normal food?

Although this strategy seems to work occasionally for adults (see Chapter 4), the answer for children in most cases seems to be no. This issue was explored in a study in which 50 children with Crohn's disease were randomly assigned to six weeks of treatment with either total enteral nutrition (24 children) or partial enteral nutrition (26 children). The children in the partial enteral nutrition group received enough of the formula to provide 50% of their estimated daily calorie requirement, and were encouraged to eat an unrestricted normal diet as well.

Only 15% of the children in the partial enteral nutrition group (4 of 26), compared with 42% of those in the total enteral nutrition group (10 of 24), achieved remission, even though the two treatments were equally effective at increasing weight and other measures of nutritional status. Measures of disease activity (hemoglobin and albumin levels, platelet count, and erythrocyte sedimentation rate) improved significantly only in the children who received total enteral nutrition, suggesting that partial enteral nutrition wasn't enough to suppress intestinal inflammation.[169]

Other studies testing supplemental enteral feeding have also reported improved growth but not reduced inflammation. In eight adolescents who received nightly supplements (1,000 to 1,500 calories per night), average growth increased from ½" to 2¾" per year, but disease activity was unchanged.[170] Likewise, in six adolescent boys, nightly supplements increased average growth from less than ¹⁄₁₆" per month to ⅕" per month, similar to the growth rate of healthy teenagers. But mild chronic disease activity continued.[171]

❖ **Total enteral nutrition is most effective at inducing remission, even though supplemental enteral nutrition can improve growth and help maintain remission.**

## Diana's Story

Diana was diagnosed with ileocolonic Crohn's disease, gastritis, and esophagitis at the age of 12. She had been in the 50th to 75th percentile for height and weight as a young child, but had dropped to the 3rd percentile by the time of her diagnosis. Her parents chose to start Diana on an enteral nutrition formula (Modulen IBD) as the initial treatment for her disease. Her mother, Lisa describes the reasons for the decision and the results:

"When we got the dreaded diagnosis, I wanted to avoid prednisone for Diana for several reasons. 1) I wanted to optimize her growth. 2) Her bone density was already low and I didn't want to make it worse with steroids. 3) Most importantly, I didn't want to put her psychological health in jeopardy. We were already dealing with depression/anxiety issues as well as ADHD [attention-deficit hyperactive disorder] and I wanted to keep her in the best mental health she was capable of.

"Enteral nutrition seemed to fit the bill for what we needed to induce remission. We wouldn't have to deal with mood swings, insomnia, and all of the other host of side effects of prednisone and, as a bonus, we would be giving her body everything it needed to grow in the few years she had left to do so. So we started Diana on Modulen exclusively for six weeks. She drank what she could and what she couldn't, she got from a nasogastric tube she inserted at night and pulled out in the morning. Meanwhile, she started on Pentasa and azathioprine to maintain remission. The first round of Modulen went well although it was difficult for Diana to not eat, especially around Thanksgiving. Fortunately a growth spurt showed her that her body did indeed need the nutrition she was getting. Her body was clearly responding to the increased nutrition.

"After the initial six weeks were up, we kept her on supplemental nocturnal feedings and she maintained remission that way for several months. When she completely stopped, however, the disease reared its ugly head. We had not yet gotten a therapeutic 6-MP level established [6-MP is the active component of azathioprine], so we did another six weeks of exclusive. This time it only kept her in remission for a week following reintroduction of food. We have not yet been able to keep her disease in remission without a significant amount of enteral nutrition and we still don't have therapeutic 6-MP levels. It is difficult and takes a lot of discipline, but it works where nothing else has AND we have avoided prednisone. Diana is now in the 40th percentile for height and weight."

# Which children respond best to enteral nutrition?

Unfortunately, not everyone goes into remission from total enteral nutrition, even though almost every child with Crohn's can benefit from enteral nutrition supplements if he or she needs to gain height and weight. It would be very helpful to know which children are most likely to respond to total enteral nutrition, to save others from having to try it and fail.

Children with certain complications of Crohn's disease such as strictures, fistulas, and/or perianal disease may have a more difficult time achieving complete remission using enteral nutrition and tend to need longer courses of treatment. We'll learn more about these issues in Chapter 5.

There may also be a trend for children with newly diagnosed Crohn's disease to respond better to total enteral nutrition than those who have been ill for a while.[172] But so far, there isn't enough evidence to draw any firm conclusions about that. All we can say at present is that Crohn's is often easier to treat when it first appears than after someone has had it for a while, regardless of the therapy chosen.[173]

Disease location is another critical factor that may affect response. As mentioned earlier in this chapter, doctors have long suspected that Crohn's disease limited to the large intestine, also known as Crohn's colitis, responds less well to total enteral nutrition than disease affecting both the small and large intestine or confined to the small intestine alone.

In a study designed to test this issue, 65 children were treated with total enteral nutrition for eight weeks. Fourteen had Crohn's in the colon, 12 had ileal disease, and 39 were affected in both locations. Only 50% of the children with Crohn's colitis went into remission, compared with 82% of those with ileocolonic disease and 92% of those with ileal disease. Additionally, the children with ileocolonic disease had significant endoscopic and histologic improvement in the colon, whereas the children with colonic disease did not.[174]

The results of another study also suggest that disease limited to the large intestine may be least responsive to total enteral nutrition. Researchers analyzed the records of 65 children and teenagers who had been treated with total enteral nutrition for an average of one and a half months. Although 72% achieved remission, success rates depended on disease location. Those with Crohn's colitis were least likely to reach remission (1 of 5, 20%), compared with over 70% of the 33 with ileocolonic disease and approximately 80% of the 27 with small bowel disease.[175]

In contrast, a couple of other retrospective studies didn't find that disease location affected the likelihood of achieving remission.[176] But at least two suggested that the disease site influenced the length of time the children *remained* in remission. In one, average length of remission was 16.4 months after treating small intestinal disease with total enteral nutrition, 5.3 months after treating ileo-colonic disease, and 3.8 months after treating colonic disease.[177] In the other, the median time to relapse after a course of enteral nutrition was 22 weeks for kids with Crohn's colitis, 58 weeks for those with both small and large intestinal disease, and 104 weeks for those with disease limited to the esophagus, stomach, and small intestine.[178]

However, these differences were not statistically significant (that is, they might have occurred by chance), and it's not clear how much weight we should put on them. A randomized study comparing total enteral nutrition with steroids came to the opposite conclusion. The median length of remission after enteral nutrition was 13 months in four patients with Crohn's colitis, compared with only 5 months in eight children whose disease was not limited to the colon.[179]

Overall, the results are mixed, especially on whether disease location affects *length* of remission, but it does seem that Crohn's colitis is somewhat less responsive to total enteral nutrition than other forms of Crohn's disease. However, the data do not indicate that children with Crohn's colitis will *never* go into remission from total enteral nutrition. There are plenty of cases that prove the contrary.[180] The data simply imply that the odds for success may be less than for children with Crohn's colitis than for those with other patterns of disease.

## What do children think about enteral nutrition?

There aren't a lot of studies of how children feel about using enteral nutrition. Based on the limited evidence available, most seem to prefer enteral nutrition to steroid treatment or consider the two therapies equally tolerable. For instance, in one small study, 7 of 12 kids treated with enteral nutrition disliked the taste and not having a normal diet. But of six who had experienced both enteral nutrition and steroids, four thought that the liquid diet was much better than steroids while only two considered it much worse.[181]

Among a larger group of 44 children who had experience with steroids and taking enteral nutrition through a nasogastric tube, 20 (45%) preferred the nutritional therapy, 12 (27%) favored prednisone, and the remaining 12 didn't have a preference.[182]

In another study, 51 adolescents who were using or had recently used enteral nutrition or corticosteroids participated in interviews or filled out a questionnaire about their experiences. The 25 teens who had taken steroids tended to be less satisfied with their treatment. The majority were unhappy with the weight gain and round face caused by the drug, and among 10 who were interviewed in person, 7 complained of having been verbally abused or teased by others because of their appearance. Six of the 10 were ashamed of the way their body looked.

But enteral nutrition, used by 26 of the kids, was not an easy treatment either. Although almost none of the children were hungry during treatment, most had food cravings, and approximately three-quarters avoided meals with others, including family. All but one used a nasogastric tube that remained in place twenty-four hours per day (the exception was a child who was fed nightly but removed the tube during the day). Of the 25 who used the tube continuously, 15 (60%) disliked the fact that others stared at them, to the point that one stopped going to school for four months. Most had to give up sports and couldn't sleep over at friends' houses, and the treatment also caused difficulties with taking vacations.[183]

A third study with more positive results evaluated quality of life in 26 children who received total enteral nutrition for eight weeks. All but three of them took the formula orally. In spite of the restricted diet, their scores on a quality-of-life scale improved significantly between the beginning and end of the study. The fact that 23 of the 26 children reached remission doubtless played a major role in the improved scores. But drinking the formula rather than using a feeding tube may have helped make the treatment more tolerable, too. Two of the three children who took the formula through a nasogastric tube had less positive feelings about enteral nutrition by the end of the study.[184]

### Pam's Story

While some kids prefer enteral nutrition to steroids, it's not for everyone. When Pam was diagnosed with Crohn's disease, she started treatment with Pentasa (mesalamine). Four months after the diagnosis, her parents encouraged her to try enteral nutrition formulas. She experimented with different types, but didn't like any of them, so compliance was an issue. Her mother Janet says, "Pam just didn't want to have anything to do with the formula—it made her feel too different, I think, and she hated the taste!"

A month later Pam was admitted to the hospital so that she could learn how to insert her own nasogastric tube. Janet reports: "That was frustrating for her, and didn't last. Pam was 16 when we tried it, and a very competitive athlete. She couldn't get enough calories without pumping during the day also, and she wasn't willing to do that any longer. . . . She was feeling better, but it wasn't working for her emotionally."

Pam had surgery instead to remove the diseased part of her ileum, ileocecal valve and part of her cecum. She has remained in remission since the operation on Pentasa, Imuran (azathioprine), an antacid, and an iron supplement.

## WHAT HAVE WE LEARNED?

❖ Total enteral nutrition is as effective as steroids in helping children with Crohn's disease achieve remission, is better than steroids at improving growth and healing intestinal inflammation, and can help steroid-dependent children discontinue steroids.

❖ Enteral nutrition supplements, used alongside regular food, can be very effective at helping children grow, and may assist in prolonging remission as well.

❖ Children who have Crohn's only in the large intestine may be less likely to respond to total enteral nutrition than those with disease limited to the small intestine or located in both the small and large intestines. However, some children with Crohn's colitis do well on enteral nutrition.

❖ There haven't been many studies about how children feel about using enteral nutrition, but those available suggest that most kids, but not all, consider it better than or equal to using steroids.

The next chapter explores enteral nutrition in adults with Crohn's disease. You will find much useful information in it that is also relevant to children. Or if you prefer, skip directly to Chapter 5, which addresses whether enteral nutrition works in certain complications of Crohn's.

## ❖ 4 ❖

# Good Stuff for Grown-Ups, Too!

## Enteral Nutrition for Adults

*Let your food be your medicine, and your medicine your food.*
**Hippocrates**

The odds are good that if you're an adult with Crohn's, your GI has never suggested that you try enteral nutrition. Gastroenterologists who treat adult patients, especially those in the United States, rarely see this therapy used during their training and don't think to offer it to their patients. So it's not surprising that most people with Crohn's don't know what enteral nutrition is. Yet studies and case reports published in medical journals over the last four decades show that enteral nutrition can be effective in adults of all ages. In this chapter we examine the evidence they provide. We'll discover that:

- Total enteral nutrition can induce remission in adults in as little as two weeks.
- Adding enteral nutrition supplements to a normal diet can make remission last longer.
- Enteral nutrition can help adults discontinue steroids without relapsing.
- It can induce remission in people who don't respond to steroids.

- It can heal ulcerations and reduce inflammation in the intestines.
- It can be a safe treatment option during pregnancy.

## How effective is enteral nutrition in adults?

In the following six studies, adults with active Crohn's disease were treated with total enteral nutrition:

- Thirteen adults were treated with total enteral nutrition for four weeks and six (46%) went into remission.[185]
- One hundred and thirty-six were treated for two weeks and 78 (57%) went into remission.[186]
- Ten were treated for four weeks and six (60%) went into remission.[187]
- Sixteen were treated for four weeks and 10 (63%) went into remission.[188]
- Twenty-eight were treated for four weeks and 20 (71%) went into remission.[189]
- Thirteen were treated for four weeks and 11 (85%) went into remission.[190]

The size of the studies and the success of enteral nutrition varied considerably. *But even in the study with the very worst results, almost half of the patients (46%) reached remission.*

In the largest study, the one with 136 patients, 57% achieved remission in spite of the fact that over 30% of the patients refused to stick with the diet for more than seven days. (Among those who completed the planned two weeks of treatment, 84% achieved remission.)

In another big study, 97 (84%) of 116 participants who complied well with enteral nutrition were in remission after approximately 100 days of treatment.[191]

# How does enteral nutrition compare with steroids?

One of the best ways to figure out how well a treatment for Crohn's works is to compare it with steroids. In spite of their unpleasant side effects (weight gain, insomnia, emotional upset, etc.), systemic steroids such as prednisone and prednisolone are very likely to induce at least temporary remission. For that reason, once researchers noticed that enteral nutrition seemed to help people with Crohn's, they conducted randomized studies to compare it directly with steroids.

In three such studies, each including anywhere from 21 to 32 adults, the patients who received steroids (prednisone or prednisolone) and those who received enteral nutrition were *equally likely* to reach remission.[192] In another study of similar size, the likelihood of reaching remission was significantly *better* with the nutritional treatment than with the steroid.[193] Remission rates with enteral nutrition in these four trials ranged from 67% to 80%.

So is total enteral nutrition just as effective as steroids, as the data from these trials suggests?

*Unfortunately, probably not.* Because it can be difficult to comply with enteral nutrition (many of us find it difficult to stick with dietary changes!), patients often do best in small studies in which they get a lot of personal encouragement to continue with the regimen.

In addition, when doctors need to recruit only a small number of patients for a trial, they may unconsciously offer especially strong encouragement to participate to patients they think will respond to the treatment.

As study size increases, the success rate of enteral nutrition tends to decrease. In a randomized study comparing enteral nutrition and prednisolone in 42 people, the remission rate was significantly higher with the steroid than the liquid diet (85% vs. 45%).

But nine of the 22 patients assigned to the enteral nutrition group were unwilling to comply with the treatment. Of those who did stick to the diet, 77% reached remission.[194]

## The case against enteral nutrition

Large randomized trials provide the best picture of how well a given therapy will succeed in the real world, where not every patient is highly motivated and some have disease characteristics that may be less responsive to the treatment being tested.

In the two biggest randomized studies of total enteral nutrition in adults, the nutritional treatment was compared with a two-drug treatment—a steroid (6-methylprednisolone) plus sulfasalazine. *The steroid/sulfasalazine combination was significantly more effective than enteral nutrition in both trials.* Given those results, some doctors think it's a waste of time to offer enteral nutrition to adults. But let's take a closer look at the two studies and see whether such pessimism is really justified.

The first trial included 95 adults with Crohn's. After six weeks of treatment, 41% of those using enteral nutrition were in remission, compared with 73% of those taking the steroid/sulfasalazine combination, a significant difference.[195]

But compliance was a *big* problem in this trial. Among the patients assigned to use enteral nutrition, 20 quit because they disliked the diet—10 wouldn't even continue beyond the first few days of treatment. So we have to wonder if more of these patients would have reached remission if they had been willing to drink the formula.

That unanswered question prompted researchers to carry out a second six-week trial comparing enteral nutrition with the same combination of medications in 107 adults. This time the patients were given the formula through a feeding tube so they wouldn't have to taste it. (See Chapter 8 for more information about tube feeding.)

Among those who received enteral nutrition, 53% reached remission, compared with 79% of those who received steroid/sulfasalazine treatment—again, a significant difference.[196] But the results for enteral nutrition were better in this trial than the prior one, probably due primarily to better compliance. Only 7 patients refused to continue with the diet, compared with 20 in the earlier study.

The steroid/sulfasalazine combination was the most effective treatment in both of these trials, *but . . .* the results do not suggest that enteral nutrition is ineffective. When patients with Crohn's disease receive placebos (substances without any actual therapeutic affect), anywhere from zero to 28% of them are likely to reach remission in two to twelve weeks.[197] Remission rates with enteral nutrition were well above that placebo level in both of these trials (41% and 53%), in spite of the problems with compliance.

In other words, enteral nutrition might not have been as effective as the steroid/sulfasalazine duo, but it put considerably more patients into remission than we would expect a placebo to do. Plus, those who did reach remission with enteral nutrition improved just as much as their fellow patients who reached remission with steroids.

Although on average fewer adults will respond to enteral nutrition than to a combination of sulfasalazine and a steroid, some people look at the advantages of enteral nutrition and make it their first option, keeping medications in reserve if the nutritional treatment doesn't work.

"After detailed discussion [nutritional support] may be used in preference to steroids, immunomodulators, or surgery for any patient with active disease, or for those unresponsive to mesalazine or in whom corticosteroids are contraindicated."
*Guidelines for the Management of Inflammatory Bowel Disease in Adults, IBD Section of the British Society of Gastroenterology* [198]

# Enteral nutrition can work when steroids do not

Enteral nutrition can be a particularly good option for people who don't respond (or no longer respond) to steroids. You might want to consider enteral nutrition if you are:

- **steroid-dependent** (can't taper and withdraw corticosteroid therapy without relapsing), or
- **steroid-refractory** (don't go into remission even if you take steroids).

One study of enteral nutrition included 5 patients who were steroid-dependent and 11 who were steroid-refractory. This group of patients presented a real challenge to their doctors. Those who were steroid-dependent had been taking prednisolone for anywhere from 18 months to 12 years. They relapsed whenever it was discontinued. Those who were steroid-refractory all had active disease in spite of daily prednisolone use. After beginning total enteral nutrition:

- Ten patients (63%) were in remission and off steroids in just four weeks.
- Seven remained in remission without any medication for at least six months.
- Three were still in remission after 18 to 32 months.[199]

Another study showed similar benefits. Eighteen adults with steroid-dependent or steroid-refractory Crohn's were treated with enteral nutrition for anywhere from 20 to 74 days (most often for about a month). Out of 20 courses of treatment (two of the patients were treated a second time after achieving some months of remission and then relapsing), eleven courses (61%) resulted in steroid-free remission.[200]

In a third study, three of seven patients with steroid-dependent Crohn's reached steroid-free remission thanks to total enteral nutrition.[201]

Enteral nutrition even works for people who have been on steroids for many months. Five of 18 adults on steroids were able to discontinue them completely after up to eight weeks of total enteral nutrition—even though they had been dependent on prednisone for an average of three and a half years![202]

## Endoscopies and biopsies prove that enteral nutrition works

Enteral nutrition can heal ulcerations affecting the **intestinal mucosa** (lining of the intestines)—something that steroids rarely do. The proof comes from studies in which doctors looked inside the intestines using x-rays or an **endoscope** (a tube with a camera attached to the end). Sometimes they also took **biopsies** (samples of intestinal tissue) and examined them under a microscope to assess healing.

In one of these studies, x-rays taken before and after treatment showed significant improvement in the intestinal mucosa of adults who received six weeks of treatment with total enteral nutrition. There wasn't any mucosal improvement in patients who received prednisolone for the same time period. Then the patients who had received the steroid were given enteral nutrition instead. After four weeks of the nutritional treatment, x-rays showed that most of them had improved, too.[203]

There's more:

- Among 28 adults who used total enteral nutrition for four weeks, approximately three-quarters had at least some **endoscopic improvement** (that is, healing seen through an endoscope) in the terminal ileum and/or the large intestine. Over half had biopsy-proven improvement.[204]

- Major endoscopic improvement was observed in 12 of 24 patients who had colonoscopies before and after a 22- to 43-day course of total enteral nutrition.[205]
- Of 10 patients who agreed to have a colonoscopy after four weeks of total enteral nutrition, 3 had total or subtotal healing of intestinal lesions.[206]

Would every trace of intestinal damage, right down to the microscopic level, heal completely if you stuck with total enteral nutrition for long enough? Possibly in some people, but probably not in all. Some people respond better to enteral nutrition than others, just as response differs with every other treatment.

## Supplemental enteral nutrition: the easiest way to better health

Not everyone is willing to give up their usual meals to try total enteral nutrition, no matter how good the potential benefits might be. Luckily, there is an easier option that can offer many of the same benefits: **supplemental enteral nutrition**. Using supplemental enteral nutrition means that you continue eating your normal diet, but consume some enteral nutrition as well. It's a way of benefiting from enteral nutrition *without* giving up your favorite foods.

Even small amounts of supplemental enteral nutrition can make a difference. If your Crohn's disease is active and you're losing weight, adding around 500 to 600 calories per day of an enteral nutrition formula to your regular diet can help put the pounds back on.[207]

Although supplementing at this level doesn't seem to have much effect on disease activity, reversing weight loss is still a big deal. Getting back to your ideal weight can make a tremendous difference in the amount of energy you have on a day-to-day basis. Being properly nourished makes it easier to fight off illness, too, and to withstand surgery, if you ever need to have it.

"In the presence of malnutrition (whether generalized undernour-ishment or a specific deficiency), supplementation with a defined-formula diet (around 500 ml per day) is recommended." *

*Guidelines of the German Society of Digestive and Metabolic Diseases*[208]

*500 ml is approximately 17 fluid ounces—just over two cups—in US measures.

## Maintaining remission with supplemental enteral nutrition

Consuming just a little more enteral nutrition can help prevent a relapse. In a study of this tactic, 39 patients with Crohn's in remission chose between using enteral nutrition along with their regular diet for a year or continuing without supplementation. Twenty-one opted for the supplement. They were instructed to drink enough of the formula to equal between 35% and 50% of their typical daily calorie intake, *without* reducing the amount of regular food they ate. On average, they consumed 769 calories of the supplement per day. Regardless of whether they were using the supplement, all 39 patients continued to take their usual maintenance medications, but those using steroids tried to taper them if possible.

Four patients disliked the supplement and gave it up within the first two weeks. But of the remaining 17, 10 (59%) were still in remission after 12 months! Eight of the 10 were steroid-free, and the other 2 were taking only a 2-mg daily dose.

In contrast, only 4 (22%) of the 18 patients who didn't supplement were in remission after one year.[209]

### Dav1d's Story

Dav1d, who is 50 years old (and proud of his unique first name!), has used enteral nutrition supplements for years. "Enteral nutrition," he says, "combined with occasional surgery and good health management has allowed me to get where I am today: healthy and happy." He reports:

"My Crohn's disease diagnosis came in the operating room of my local Toronto hospital in 1973. Obviously, I had Crohn's before that diagnosis, but until I had an acute episode with a complete blockage requiring surgery, no one called it Crohn's. For me, that was the beginning of a new phase of my life. I went from being a small, thin, often sick kid to an in-the-hospital and out-of-the-hospital teenager and then adult. People no longer asked about school or sports, it was always 'How's your health today?' Since then, I've had four major surgeries (resections), and a number of smaller procedures (e.g., fistulae), and a few hospitalizations for poor health, including dehydration and rapid loss of weight.

"So I've had all kinds of supplemental nutrition over the years. And most of that was enteral nutrition. TPN was the mechanism of choice only for the major surgeries, where total bowel rest was required. It's the tube feedings and twenty-five years of Ensure Plus Strawberry ('EPS') that has really kept me going. I still drink three to four cans of EPS every day, but I am eating a full diet as well. I try and put in 3,000+ calories a day. And I'm doing it! I've put on a bit of weight (approximately 10 pounds) in the last few months. And I've been almost symptom-free for 10 years.

"But times weren't always as good as they are now. There was a point when my GI doctor told me I needed surgery, and I simply refused to submit. My life was too busy to carve out a recovery schedule. I was not supposed to eat solid food because of the internal leakage, so my diet was limited to clear liquids and EPS. I thought I could live the rest of my life on EPS and clear liquids. I started leaving cans of EPS in friends' fridges so I'd always have access to 'a cold one.' I used the fridge at work. I carried a cooler in my car that was always plugged into the power socket to keep the drinks cold. Even when I traveled, I could always find EPS in the local pharmacies (including Hawaii, Amsterdam, and Israel!). But after 444 days (yeah, you read that correctly—more than one year), I realized that I couldn't postpone that surgery forever. During that 444-day, no-solid-food period, I had to go through two Christmas seasons, two Passover feasts, uncounted family dinners, client lunches, power breakfasts, and dinner dates with women. I drank between ten and twelve cans of EPS per day, every single day. (I did cheat with semisolid food on a few occasions, and paid dearly for it for the following two days, but each incident was a calculated gambit based on events on my personal-life calendar.)

"The surgery went well, and I went back to a solid diet with EPS as a supplement (at least three cans per day). Throughout the past 35 years, Crohn's hasn't slowed me down (except during acute attacks). I am an enterpreneur, have started a number of successful small businesses, own two cars, one small condominium, and a four-seat airplane. And . . . I love life."

## Getting off steroids with supplemental enteral nutrition

Another study of supplementing enrolled 33 patients with Crohn's who were all in remission on steroids, but relapsed whenever they tried to taper and withdraw the medication. They were advised to drink enough of an enteral nutrition formula to equal 35% of their typical daily calorie intake, without reducing their normal food consumption.

Six people gave up on the treatment within the first two weeks because they disliked using the formula. But sticking with the therapy paid off for others. Of the 27 who continued to supplement, 19 (70%) were able to discontinue prednisone without relapsing. Fourteen of them stayed in remission for at least 12 months and the remaining five for at least 6 months.

After completing the original one-year study protocol, the 14 patients who were still in remission were given the choice of continuing nutritional supplementation for another 12 months or discontinuing it. Of seven who quit using their supplement, all relapsed within four months and had to restart steroids. But among the seven who continued supplementation, six were still in remission and off steroids at the end of 24 months.[210]

❖ **If supplementing works for you, and you're willing to stick with it, it can make a real difference in keeping you in remission.**

## Getting into remission with supplemental enteral nutrition

Some people are even able to induce remission by doing nothing except adding enteral nutrition supplements to their regular diet. In a study testing this approach, 11 patients who failed to respond to high-dose steroids were placed on a very high-calorie diet—100 calories for every kilogram (2.2 pounds) of ideal body weight. That would work out to 5,700 calories per day for a woman whose normal weight should be 125 pounds (57 kilograms), or 7,300 calories per day for a man who should weigh 160 pounds (77 kilograms). Half of the calories came from nightly tube feeding with an enteral nutrition formula and the other half from a low-residue diet.

By the end of the first week of the study, the patients were consuming an average of 5,855 calories per day through this combination of enteral nutrition and regular food. Although they only continued with the regimen for an average of 20 days, 8 of the 11 patients achieved remission, and the average length of remission was six months. Patients with **strictures** (narrowed areas of intestine) were able to eat foods that previously caused subacute obstruction by the time that they had completed only one week of treatment.[211]

# Supplementing: is more better than less?

In the studies of supplemental enteral nutrition we've looked at so far, enteral nutrition was *added* to a normal diet. A more rigorous method of supplementing involves *replacing* one or two meals per day with enteral nutrition. This approach has been tested in Japan, where supplemental enteral nutrition is a standard maintenance therapy for Crohn's.

In several of the Japanese studies, patients were asked to get 50% or more of their calories from night-time tube feeding with an elemental diet and the remainder from one or two low-fat meals eaten during the day. Compared with patients following an unsupplemented, unrestricted diet, the patients who supplemented achieved:

- significantly lower relapse rates
- significantly reduced likelihood of endoscopic recurrence
- significantly lower concentrations of inflammation-causing cytokines (small proteins produced by the immune system).[212]

Retrospective studies suggest that this type of supplementation may prevent or at least delay the need for an intestinal resection.[213] Also, consuming 1,200 calories or more per day of enteral nutrition may be better than lower levels of consumption.[214]

Twenty-two patients who used enteral nutrition to supply more than two-thirds of their daily calories achieved particularly impressive results. Their remaining calories came from low-residue solid food, and they limited their fat consumption to less than 15 grams per day and restricted their consumption of meat. *They had a cumulative rate of continuous remission of 94% after one year, 63% after two years, and 63% after four years.*[215]

However, these patients, as well as most of the others participating in the studies described in this section, were not randomly assigned to enteral nutrition or an unrestricted diet. That makes it hard to tell whether the participants who used considerable quantities of enteral nutrition differed from those who didn't in characteristics that could affect their health. They might have been more committed to maintaining a healthy lifestyle or might have responded better to enteral nutrition than those who gave it up quickly or chose not to use it.

We also don't know whether restricting regular food intake to low-fat and low-residue items improves the success of supplemental enteral nutrition compared with supplementing an unrestricted diet. But at a minimum, it's clear that people whose disease responds well to enteral nutrition can benefit from supplementing, whatever regimen they choose to adopt.

## Who responds best to enteral nutrition?

Even among those who are willing to stick with total enteral nutrition or substantial amounts of supplemental enteral nutrition, not all will go into or remain in remission. People with strictures, fistulas, and/or perianal disease may have a more difficult time achieving full remission with enteral nutrition, and tend to need longer courses of treatment. We'll learn more about these issues in Chapter 5.

In addition, some studies suggest that people who have **Crohn's colitis** (Crohn's disease limited to the colon) or substantial colonic involvement accompanying small intestinal disease may be somewhat less likely to respond to enteral nutrition than those with disease limited to the small intestine.[216] People in these categories may also be quicker to relapse after reaching remission.[217]

Finally, patients who had Crohn's disease for a long time may not be quite as apt to respond to enteral nutrition as those with new-onset disease.[218]

But the evidence for all these generalizations is mixed. In one series of 87 patients who received enteral nutrition, those who failed to improve were significantly more likely to have severe disease activity, bleeding, marked colonic involvement, and long-standing disease.[219] But in another series of 113 patients, the success of enteral nutrition wasn't affected by disease location, level of disease activity, the patient's sex or age, or whether the disease was newly diagnosed or long-standing.[220]

There is insufficient evidence from *any* of the available studies of adults to offer conclusive findings on which patients respond best, although assessed in conjunction with the data from studies of children (see Chapter 3), it is probably fair to conclude that Crohn's colitis, at least, is not as responsive to total enteral nutrition as Crohn's in the small intestine.

Nevertheless, even having Crohn's colitis is not a reason to discard total enteral nutrition as a treatment option without trying it first. The results may surprise you. One trial of total enteral nutrition in adults that included an unusually large percentage of patients with colonic disease (20 of 30 had Crohn's colitis) nevertheless achieved a 70% remission rate.[221] Like all therapies for Crohn's, enteral nutrition works for some people and not for others, and you won't know if it's going to work for you until you try.

## A safe treatment option during pregnancy

Many women with Crohn's who are eager to have a baby worry that the medications they take could harm the fetus. If you are planning to become pregnant, and possibly to breast-feed as well, you might want to consider enteral nutrition. Because it is a food rather than a drug, there are no medication-related side effects to worry about.

Although there is still not much published information on the use of enteral nutrition by pregnant women, case reports testify to the fact that it has been used successfully to control active Crohn's disease during pregnancy.

One woman pregnant with twins was given enteral nutrition on three occasions during her pregnancy. The most sustained treatment was given during a relapse at 26 weeks. She received 12,000 calories of the formula and recovered quickly (the number of days for which she was treated is not stated).[222]

Four other women with small intestinal or ileocolonic Crohn's disease each used two-week courses of total enteral nutrition to treat one or two relapses that occurred during pregnancy. Three of them used enteral nutrition supplements to maintain remission as well. They consumed anywhere from 730 to 1,450 calories of formula per day, beginning after the first or second relapse.[223]

If you are thinking of trying enteral nutrition, you might want to test-drive it *before* becoming pregnant to see if it works for you. If it does, it could be your key to achieving to a safe and worry-free pregnancy. Check with your doctor before starting to make sure the formula you choose has all the nutrients you need while expecting. Most importantly:

❖ **If you use total enteral nutrition during pregnancy, make sure you consume enough calories to cover your own nutritional needs and those of your baby.**

## Is enteral nutrition too difficult for adults?

There are times when enteral nutrition seems to be the ideal option—when someone is worried about drug side effects, for instance, or has stopped responding to other drugs. But even then some doctors don't bother to mention enteral nutrition because they assume that patients are unlikely to comply with the diet.

This is not an unjustified concern. As we have seen, some trials of enteral nutrition in adults had high dropout rates. A certain proportion of people who try enteral nutrition, even those who are only using enteral nutrition supplements, refuse to continue after a day or two. They find it too difficult to give up their normal eating habits, regardless of the potential benefit.

This lack of compliance tends to discourage doctors, even those who are initially enthusiastic about enteral nutrition. Think about the situation from your gastroenterologist's point of view. It can be time-consuming to explain the treatment, help a patient get samples of different formulas to try, fight for insurance coverage of the formula, and arrange for equipment and training if an individual chooses tube feeding rather than drinking the diet. Then if the patient quits taking the formula before giving it a chance to work, all the time expended is wasted. A doctor who has gone through that is less likely to offer enteral nutrition to the next patient who comes along.

But even in the randomized study of enteral nutrition with the worst compliance (41% of the participants quit), more than half of the patients *didn't* give up.[224] Just because *some* adults find the treatment too difficult doesn't mean that enteral nutrition should be abandoned entirely. There are people who prefer enteral nutrition to any other therapy.

When adults who had used total enteral nutrition at least once were asked whether they would prefer to treat their next relapse of Crohn's with enteral nutrition or "other medical treatment," 65% said they would prefer enteral nutrition![225]

Might you be one of them? The only way to find out is to try it and see. (In Chapter 8 you'll find some tips for successfully completing a course of enteral nutrition.)

### Sharon's Story

Sharon, the mother of an 18-year-old with Crohn's, says, "Even in the UK we have faced doctors saying 'Well, okay, it's all right for you, but it's much too hard for other families.' I spoke to one mother with a daughter whose sight was in danger due to a steroid reaction and her doctors had told her that [enteral nutrition] would work but that it would be too hard. My GI sent me to talk to her on the basis that how hard is the choice between losing your sight and not doing so, and in the process gaining remission!"

## WHAT HAVE WE LEARNED?

❖ Total enteral nutrition tends to be less effective than steroids in adults with Crohn's, but remission rates still range between 41% and 85%. It can be effective in patients who don't respond to steroids or no longer respond to them, and is more effective than steroids at healing the lining of the intestines.

❖ Using small quantities of enteral nutrition supplements (500 or 600 calories per day) in addition to a normal diet can help malnourished patients gain weight and correct nutritional deficiencies. Using larger amounts of supplements in addition to a normal diet, or in place of one or two of meals per day, can help patients reduce steroid use and maintain remission.

❖ People with Crohn's colitis may be less likely to respond to enteral nutrition than those with Crohn's in the small intestine, and patients with long-term disease may be a little less likely to respond than those with new-onset disease. However, many patients in both categories can still use enteral nutrition successfully.

In the next chapter, we will learn about some specific complications of Crohn's and discover whether they can be treated with enteral nutrition.

## ❖ 5 ❖

# Time for a Challenge

## Enteral Nutrition in Complicated Crohn's

Why is it when everyone feasts on the
pleasures of life, I get the indigestion?
**Dennis the Menace (1993)**

If you have lived with Crohn's for any length of time, you know
that the disease, or problems associated with it, can pop up virtually anywhere in the body. This chapter explores the use of enteral
nutrition to treat some of the more difficult or less common manifestations of Crohn's disease, occurring from the mouth on down. If you
have a particular complication of Crohn's disease—arthritis or a fistula, for example—and you want to know whether anyone has used
enteral nutrition to treat a similar problem, this is the place to look.

## Enteral nutrition in orofacial Crohn's

Orofacial Crohn's disease is just what its name implies: Crohn's affecting the face and the inside and outside of the mouth. If you
have Crohn's, you may be all too familiar with **aphthous ulcers**,
mouth sores that can make eating and drinking painful. In addition,
orofacial Crohn's can cause large ulcerations and unsightly swelling
involving the gums, lips, and cheeks.

Only a couple of case reports describe people who used enteral
nutrition to treat orofacial Crohn's. One patient was an eight-year-old

girl with mouth ulcers and swollen lips and gums. Her symptoms disappeared during six weeks of total enteral nutrition.[226]

Another child, a 12-year-old boy, was diagnosed with Crohn's after three months of facial swelling and a year of on-and-off diarrhea. He improved dramatically within two days of beginning enteral nutrition, and was treated with enteral nutrition for two relapses as well.[227]

Two reports aren't enough for us to estimate how often orofacial Crohn's will respond to enteral nutrition. However, they do suggest that enteral nutrition is a potential treatment option if you are suffering from orofacial disease.

## Treating fistulas with enteral nutrition

**Fistulas** are abnormal passages that open up between areas of the body that would not normally be connected. Some common types of fistulas that can occur people with Crohn's include:

- enterocutaneous fistulas (connecting a section of intestines with the skin)
- enteroenteric fistulas (connecting one loop of intestine with another)
- enterovesical fistulas (connecting an area of the intestines with the bladder)
- enterovaginal fistulas (linking the rectum or colon and the vagina)
- perianal fistulas (fistulas having their outlets in the anal area or perineal region).

A big clue that a fistula is present is when feces begins to show up in the wrong place. For instance, stool can leak into the vagina from an opening in the **rectum** (the area of the large intestine where stool is stored) or **colon** (the longest part of the large intestine) if you have an enterovaginal fistula. It can show up in urine if you have an enterovesical fistula because the fistula allows feces to pass from the intestines to the bladder.

Fistulas are a challenge for enteral nutrition. They tend to be slow to respond, some remaining unchanged after three to five weeks of treatment. Others will close or begin to drain less within this time span, although they are likely to recur within weeks or months of resuming a normal diet.[228]

Those who stick with enteral nutrition for as much as three or four months have the best odds of achieving fistula closure. The strongest evidence for this comes from a study of 68 men and women who had a total of 75 fistulas that weren't draining very heavily (they were treated promptly before they worsened).[229] Most of the fistulas (45 of them) were perianal, but there were also twelve enterocutaneous fistulas, six enteroenteric, four enterovesical, four enterovaginal, and four internal fistulas with abscesses.

After an average of 101 days of total enteral nutrition, 54 of the 75 fistulas (72%) had closed and 20 (15%) were partially closed, leaving only six that didn't respond at all. Enterocutaneous fistulas were quickest to close, requiring about 23 days of treatment, compared with around 50 days for enteroenteric, enterovesical, and enterovaginal fistulas. Healing time is not stated for the perianal fistulas.

Unfortunately, this study doesn't provide any details on the crucial issue of how long the fistulas *stayed* closed. But the few published cases reporting long-term success with fistula closure almost all describe patients who continued to use enteral nutrition for substantial periods of time.

- A woman with fistulas around the anus and vulva achieved long-term fistula closure thanks to an 11-week course of total enteral nutrition.[230]

- An enterocutaneous fistula closed in a patient who supplemented his diet with enteral nutrition four nights per week (1,700 calories per night). He remained on this regimen and the fistula was still closed five months later.[231]

- A child had a perianal fistula and perianal ulcer that had persisted for three years in spite of treatment with steroids and sulfa drugs. They closed during ten weeks of total enteral nutrition and did not return when the boy resumed his regular diet.[232]

There is also a report of an enterocutaneous fistula that closed during four weeks of total enteral nutrition and was still closed over a year later.[233]

Still, evidence for long-term fistula closure remains meager. The odds are reasonably good that you can achieve fistula closure if you continue total enteral nutrition for three or four months, but there is no guarantee that the fistula will stay closed after you return to your normal diet. Also, the occasional patient has a very poor response: the fistula may increase in size, with enteral nutrition appearing to drain directly from it.[234] Thus enteral nutrition is not the ideal treatment for fistulas—but unfortunately nothing is.

It is difficult to achieve and maintain fistula closure on a long-term basis regardless of the therapy you choose. Surgery, antibiotics, immunomodulators, biologics—all work in some cases, but often only temporarily, and none are foolproof. Enteral nutrition is one more treatment option to consider.

## Enteral nutrition in perianal disease

Perianal disease refers to Crohn's symptoms affecting the skin around the anal and perineal area, including **fissures** (tears in the skin), fistulas, and ulcers. Treating perianal disease with enteral nutrition demands considerable patience.

In a small study of total enteral nutrition in children, fissures improved relatively quickly, but anorectal fistulas healed slowly over a matter of months.[235]

In adults treated with total enteral nutrition for about a month, six patients had reduced output from perianal fistulas, but only one patient had a perianal fistula that closed.[236] In another study, perianal fistulas in two children failed to close during three weeks of total enteral nutrition.[237]

In two adults, rectal fissures and perianal ulcerations healed after two to three weeks of total enteral nutrition. However, these patients did not have fistulas in the perianal region, which take longer to respond than fissures and ulcers.[238] Fistulas and, to a lesser extent, anal lesions, were the complications most likely to reduce the probability of reaching remission in a study of 139 patients treated with enteral nutrition.[239]

Even when perianal disease responds to enteral nutrition, it may recur quickly. Nine of 12 adults with perianal disease reached remission on total enteral nutrition in one study, but all but one relapsed within eight weeks of returning to a normal diet. Also, the perianal complications responded much more slowly to enteral nutrition than the patients' other intestinal symptoms.[240]

All in all, perianal disease is among the tougher complications of Crohn's disease to treat with enteral feeding. Success is possible, but not guaranteed, and may be difficult to maintain after returning to regular food. Nevertheless, enteral nutrition is worth remembering if nothing else is available or nothing else works.

### Daniel's Story

As a boy, Daniel, now 18, had Crohn's throughout the entire intestinal tract, from mouth to anus. He didn't respond to standard drug treatments (budesonide, prednisolone, azathiaprine), nor to a polymeric enteral nutrition formula, Modulen IBD. His mother, Sharon, reports:

"Along the way he had also aquired a large and many-tracted perianal fistula that we treated with Flagyl [metronidazole], but it had remained open. Our doctors were reluctant to operate as the result would be uncertain, to say the least. Medical opinion was that it wouldn't close, but that we should just put off dealing with it until his condition became more stable. At this point our only other option was Remicade. We knew his terminal ileum was strictured and we wanted to avoid Remicade as the likely result would have been immediate surgery for the stricture.

"As a last ditch before Remicade we tried an elemental formula, Elemental EO28, and bingo, three weeks later he was in clinical remission for the first time, and in the next three weeks grew 1½". Since then he has followed a regime using overnight feeds to maintain remission and periods of exclusive (usually six weeks) when he needs to—three to four times a year. His fisula closed . . . and an MRI scan shows no trace. I guess it was about a year of the mix of [supplementing and exclusive enteral nutrition] that did the trick, with about four bouts of exclusive. The only explanation is that the prolonged use allowed his body to heal. He is planning to continue this treatment as an adult basically because it is the only thing we know that works."

Daniel ultimately did have a resection and a stricturoplasty to treat the strictures he developed before starting enteral nutrition. But by then, Sharon says, the elemental formula "had done its magic on his gut and the surgeon said he was amazed after the results of his previous scopes, etc., in what good shape his gut was in. He lost so little [intestine] that that there are no long-term nutritional issues for him."

## Strictures and enteral nutrition

A **stricture**, also called a **stenosis** (plural: **stenoses**), is an area where the intestinal tract has narrowed, making it is difficult for food to pass through. Food caught in a stricture can cause partial or complete intestinal obstruction.

There are two main types of strictures that occur in patients with Crohn's. The first type is caused by acute inflammation. If the walls of the intestine are inflamed, the swelling can make the passage of food difficult. With treatment of Crohn's disease that reduces inflammation, this type of stricture may disappear.

If there is long-term inflammation or repeated cycles of inflammation, scarring builds up and strictures can become thick, fibrous, and permanent.

The response of strictures to enteral nutrition is uneven. There are reports of strictures that remained unchanged after six months, nine months, or even fifteen months of enteral nutrition, although the patients otherwise went into remission and were totally symptom-free as long as they stuck to a liquid diet.[241]

On the other hand, total enteral nutrition has been used to successfully treat an ureteral obstruction, two cecal strictures, and two duodenal strictures (including one that had not responded to TPN).[242] Enteral nutrition also markedly improved an ileal stricture and reduced multiple inflammatory masses to isolated stenoses.[243]

Why was enteral nutrition successful in some cases and not others? Response seems to depend on two main factors. The first is treatment time. Although rapid improvement is possible (one of the duodenal strictures improved a great deal in two weeks), strictures often need several months or more of treatment. For example, in four children who used enteral nutrition, strictures were unchanged after a month, but three strictures had disappeared and the fourth had improved by the end of 12 months. (These children received total enteral nutrition for two to seven months, followed by nightly supplements supplying 50% of their calories for the remainder of the year.)[244]

The other issue that affects response is the nature of the stricture. Long-standing fibrous strictures are unlikely to respond to total enteral nutrition. Symptoms of obstruction tend to recur as soon as a patient resumes eating solid food.[245] If you suffer from such strictures, you may need a **stricturoplasty** or a **resection** (surgeries that widen or remove areas of intestine, respectively), or an **endoscopic balloon dilation** (a nonsurgical procedure to stretch open a stricture) in order to return successfully to an unrestricted diet.

❖ **Enteral nutrition can reverse inflammatory strictures, but is unlikely to change thick and fibrous strictures.**

One further consideration may be of interest to those with strictures. There is limited evidence (from a single retrospective study) that supplementing your diet with enteral nutrition after an operation to treat strictures may extend the length of remission after surgery and reduce your risk of needing another operation. In that study, about 38% of patients who consumed over 600 calories per day of an elemental diet for one or more years after surgery were still in remission five years later, compared with 29% of those who used less or no enteral nutrition.[246]

### Gail's Story

Gail was diagnosed with a stricture in the terminal ileum. She had an endoscopic balloon dilation to widen the narrowed area, but her symptoms returned in a few months. At that point she decided to try supplemental enteral nutrition. "I felt I had to walk the walk if I was going to preach this to my kids," Gail says. (She has two children with Crohn's who use enteral nutrition.)

Gail used a semi-elemental formula called Peptamen for approximately five months. She began with three cans a day, totaling 750 calories, for a month or two, then dropped to two cans a day and then one before discontinuing. The regimen was a success: "My GI says the longest he's had a dilation hold is two years. At six years out, and no surgery yet, I am the longest running holdout he's seen."

# Enteral nutrition for esophageal Crohn's

Crohn's disease in the **esophagus** (the tube running from the mouth to the stomach) can cause ulcers, strictures, and fistulas, just like Crohn's affecting other parts of the gastrointestinal tract. Only two cases have been described in which enteral nutrition was used in esophageal Crohn's. However, the results achieved were promising.

A 32-year-old woman had struggled with oral and colonic Crohn's for nine years in spite of treatment with steroids, mesalamine, and azathioprine. Ultimately she tried total enteral nutrition after developing ulcers and an ulcerated stricture in the esophagus.

She improved rapidly and her esophageal ulcers healed within a month. After staying on enteral nutrition for three months in all, she slowly reintroduced foods one at a time. Approximately nine months later, after she had returned to a normal diet, only a smooth stricture in the esophagus remained.[247]

Another patient, a 29-year-old woman, had esophageal disease with multiple ulcers as well as anal and colonic disease and vaginal ulcerations. After 5-ASA drugs, prednisolone, and azathioprine failed, she began total enteral nutrition. She used a gastrostomy tube, as did the prior patient, because swallowing was painful for her. (See Chapter 8 for information about feeding tubes.) Within a month, all her symptoms had disappeared, and her esophagus was completely healed.[248]

# Enteral nutrition after a resection

An intestinal **resection** is an operation to remove a portion of the intestines that is diseased, obstructed, or otherwise unusable. What happens if you need a resection? Sometimes only a small section of problematic intestine needs to be removed. Then you can return to a normal diet and with luck, enjoy a long remission.

Alternately you may require more extensive surgery. If a lot of intestine is removed, you may no longer be able to pass stool through the usual route of the colon, rectum, and anus. Instead, your surgeon will perform a type of surgery known as an **ostomy** to create a new opening (**stoma**) in the skin of the abdomen to allow the excretion of wastes. The remaining end of healthy intestine is brought through the intestinal wall to create the stoma.

Different types of ostomy operations are used depending on what part or parts of the intestines are removed. For instance, if much or all of the large intestine is removed, you may need an ileostomy. With an **ileostomy**, stool is excreted through a stoma opening from the **ileum** (the last section of the small intestine) to the abdomen. If the ileum is also removed, you might have a **jejunostomy**, in which the **jejunum** (middle section of the small intestine) is brought through the abdominal wall to create a stoma.

If just a portion of the colon or rectum is removed, you might have a **colostomy**, with the stoma made out of a remaining segment of colon.

## Treating short bowel syndrome with enteral nutrition

Resection of relatively large segments of the intestines can affect the absorption of food, vitamins, and minerals. Malabsorption is a particular problem when a resection involves the small intestine, the organ in which most food absorption takes place.

If large amounts of small intestine have to be removed, there may not be enough remaining intestine to fully absorb nutrients from a normal diet. This situation is called **short bowel syndrome**. Typical symptoms of short bowel syndrome include chronic diarrhea, dehydration, and malnutrition.

*In people with short bowel syndrome, enteral nutrition can be easier for the body to absorb than normal food.* One man with short bowel syndrome absorbed only 72% of the calories from the food he ate and only 55% of the nitrogen. (We need nitrogen to make protein.) In contrast, he absorbed 96% of the calories and 88% of the nitrogen from total enteral nutrition.[249]

Another man had a similar experience. When he switched from regular food to enteral nutrition, he absorbed 96% rather than 72% of calories he consumed and 88% rather than 41% of nitrogen. It was also much easier for him to absorb fats when he used total enteral nutrition. The amount of fat excreted in his stool (a sign of fat malabsorption) decreased from 55 to 2 grams per day.[250]

The improved absorption offered by enteral nutrition can be particularly important for people who have little healthy intestine left. A 51-year-old woman had lost her ileum, colon, and rectum and had only 47 inches of remaining **jejunum** (the middle section of the small intestine) after seventeen hospitalizations for Crohn's disease. Thanks to total enteral nutrition, she gained 30 pounds, reaching a normal weight. She remained on total enteral nutrition on a long-term basis, and as of three years later had not needed to be rehospitalized.[251]

Sometimes a short course of enteral nutrition can resolve temporary problems with malabsorption and allow people with short bowel syndrome to return to eating normal food. For example, a woman with Crohn's used total enteral nutrition for three weeks after her ileostomy output increased, causing leakage and skin problems around the ostomy site. Her ostomy output decreased substantially within a few days of starting enteral nutrition, and the skin surrounding the stoma healed during the second week of treatment. After the three weeks of enteral nutrition, she was able to resume a normal diet.[252]

Another woman with Crohn's had a colostomy output of over 80 ounces per day, a 24-pound weight loss, and severe abdominal pain before and during defecation in spite of long-term treatment with steroids. She used total enteral nutrition for 23 days, and then gradually reintroduced food, supplemented by the formula, during a 17-day period. Her stoma output decreased to 10 ounces per day, and she was able to discontinue the steroids as well as opiates she had taken for pain. Five months later, she was still symptom-free and had gained 10 pounds. Her stoma output remained at 10 ounces per day.[253]

## Supplemental enteral nutrition in short bowel syndrome

Don't want to completely give up food to use total enteral nutrition? Just using enteral nutrition supplements can help if you can't maintain a healthy weight after a resection. The following five cases show the potential benefits.

1. After a **proctocolectomy** (removal of the rectum and all or part of the colon) and multiple small intestinal resections, a 48-year-old man had only 63 inches of remaining small intestine. Although he was eating 3,500 calories per day, he lost 1,800 calories per day through his stoma and was 39 pounds underweight. He was able to regain and maintain almost all of the lost weight by tube feeding with 1,500 calories of enteral nutrition five nights per week. He ate a normal diet during the day. As soon as he stopped tube feeding, the weight loss began again, but he was able to maintain his weight by drinking 1,250 calories of enteral nutrition a day to supplement his regular meals.[254]

2. A 22-year-old woman who had had a proctocolectomy and many other surgeries had only 31½ inches of small intestine left. She absorbed only 25% of the calories contained in a 3,500 calorie diet, and was 42 pounds below her ideal weight. She was able to gain 15 pounds over three months by drinking 1,000 calories of enteral nutrition per day and taking an additional 1,000 calories nightly through a nasogastric tube. The

weight gain continued even after she reduced the overnight tube feeding to five nights per week.[255]

3. A 61-year-old man with short bowel syndrome was 28 pounds underweight. He began nighttime tube feeding with enteral nutrition, supplemented during the day by small, frequent, low-residue and lactose-free meals. Over the following year, he gained 22 pounds, had decreased daily stool output, regained his strength, and was able to resume his normal daily activities.[256]

4. A 49-year-old man whose colon and terminal ileum had been removed developed three separate fistulas around his mid-ileal ileostomy. He lost 22 pounds in six months, and was only eating 1,300 calories per day. He was tube-fed nightly with enteral nutrition (2,000 calories per night) and encouraged to eat normal food during the day. He immediately began to gain weight and consume more food during the day, and all three fistulas closed within 2½ weeks.[257]

5. A 35-year-old man with a history of ileal resection and **right hemicolectomy** (removal of the right portion of the colon) had a recurrent enterocutaneous fistula. He gained weight and the fistula closed up on TPN. But whenever he tried to return to normal food, he lost weight and the fistula reopened. He began tube feeding four nights per week (approximately 1,700 calories per night) to supplement his normal diet. The fistula stayed closed, he was able to leave the hospital, and was still doing well on follow-up approximately five months later.[258]

# Enteral nutrition and extraintestinal symptoms

Crohn's disease doesn't just affect our intestines, it can attack many other parts of the body. Symptoms of Crohn's that occur outside of the gastrointestinal tract are referred to as **extraintestinal symptoms**.

Some extraintestinal symptoms may respond to enteral nutrition, although there's not much published information to guide us. A few reports describe people who have used enteral nutrition to treat Crohn's-related joint pain, eye inflammation, and kidney disease.

## Joint pain

**Arthralgias** (joint pains that occur without visible inflammation) are a common extraintestinal symptom of Crohn's. They may migrate from one part of the body to another, and may be worse when Crohn's is active.

**Arthritis** is another type of joint pain that can be associated with Crohn's. Joint pain from arthritis, unlike that from arthralgias, is usually accompanied by swelling and stiffness.

Very few studies of enteral nutrition in Crohn's disease mention whether the patients had arthralgias or arthritis. A rare publication that addressed this issue was a study of 17 children who received total enteral nutrition. They had a wide range of Crohn's symptoms, including arthralgias in five cases. The joint pains went away after an average of 18 days of treatment.[259]

Another published report describes an 11-year-old who had inflammatory arthritis, fever, and abdominal pain associated with Crohn's in the ileum. The arthritis disappeared, along with the abdominal pain, within five or six days of beginning total enteral nutrition.[260]

See "Rob's Story" in Chapter 3 for the account of another child whose joint pain responded to enteral nutrition. Also, the case of an adult with eye and joint inflammation is described below.

## Eye inflammation

Three eye diseases can occur as extraintestinal symptoms of Crohn's: **uveitis**, **episcleritis**, and **scleritis**. Uveitis is inflammation of the lining of the eyeball (the uvea). It causes red eyes, pain, and blurred vision. Episcleritis is inflammation of the membrane (episclera) that covers the white part of the eye (the sclera). It may affect one or both eyes, causing redness but usually little discomfort. Scleritis, inflammation of the sclera, is a more serious condition. It can be extremely painful, and in some cases causes blindness.

A recently published report describes a 26-year-old woman with Crohn's who struggled with a variety of symptoms, including scleritis, that ultimately responded to enteral nutrition.[261] After being diagnosed with Crohn's in the ileum, she was treated with most of the standard Crohn's medications, including antibiotics, systemic steroids, budesonide, mesalamine, and azathioprine. She was started on Remicade after developing severe scleritis in the right eye and another extraintestinal complication, **erythema nodosum** (a skin disease causing tender red lumps, usually on the lower legs).

The biologic drug never fully controlled her symptoms. She developed psoriasis (a skin condition) three months later that would clear up for two or three weeks after each infusion and then return. She also developed arthritis and arthralgias, and had recurrent outbreaks of genital herpes. After 21 months of Remicade use, the scleritis returned with almost complete loss of vision.

At that point, she refused further Remicade treatment, and began total enteral nutrition instead. The rash caused by the psoriasis began to fade away after only four days on the formula. As she continued treatment, her joint pains disappeared, she had no further herpes outbreaks, and at the end of three weeks she regained her vision. After a total of five weeks of total enteral nutrition, she switched to a maintenance regimen of two regular meals per day plus two meals of enteral nutrition. More than five months after first starting the formula, she remained in perfect health on this regimen and was not taking any medications.

## Kidney disease

A very small percentage of people with Crohn's disease (around 1% to 2.5%) develop a kidney disease known as **renal amyloidosis**. The big challenge for these patients is to prevent the amyloidosis from progressing to kidney failure.

A single case has been published in which total enteral nutrition was used in managing a case of renal amyloidosis associated with Crohn's.[262] Chronic protein loss in urine is one of the main signs of renal amyloidosis. While using an elemental diet, the amount of protein excreted in this patient's urine decreased from 15.5 to less than 0.3 grams per day.

At the point the case report was written, the patient had stayed in remission on total enteral nutrition and off steroids for two years, with urinary protein excretion remaining below 0.3 grams per day.

# Enteral nutrition in transplant patients

Patients who are using immunosuppressive drugs for reasons other than IBD rarely develop Crohn's disease or ulcerative colitis. But there are exceptions. A teenage girl developed Crohn's even though she had taken immunosuppressive drugs since a heart transplant at the age of five. Her Crohn's symptoms disappeared during eight weeks of total enteral nutrition.[263] She began growing approximately 3" per year after treatment, compared with about ½" per year before treatment.

She supplemented her diet with the formula in order to maintain remission, but had two further relapses over the next 2½ years, one treated with total enteral nutrition and the other with three months of prednisolone. At age 18, 2½ years after the initial diagnosis, she was in good health eating two meals per day and using enteral nutrition as a supplement to provide her remaining calories.

She remained on azathioprine and tacrolimus to prevent transplant rejection.

## WHAT HAVE WE LEARNED?

❖ Although the published data is very limited, enteral nutrition may be a promising treatment for orofacial and esophageal Crohn's. It can improve joint pains associated with Crohn's as well. In a single published case, it reversed scleritis and healed psoriatic lesions.

❖ Enteral nutrition can close fistulas if used for long enough, but does not work in all cases. Fistulas that close may reopen after the diet is discontinued. Similarly, only some cases of perianal disease respond to enteral nutrition and perianal symptoms may recur after stopping the nutritional regimen.

❖ Enteral nutrition can heal inflammatory strictures, but does not eliminate long-established, fibrotic strictures.

❖ People with short bowel syndrome may have significantly better nutrient absorption if they use total enteral nutrition rather than regular food. They can also use enteral nutrition supplements to prevent or reverse serious weight loss and malnutrition.

❖ Enteral nutrition has been used at least once to manage renal amyloidosis associated with Crohn's, and to control Crohn's in an organ transplant patient.

In the next chapter, we'll explore the potential of enteral nutrition in treating diseases other than Crohn's. If you have already been diagnosed with Crohn's, you may want to skip directly to Chapter 7, where we'll learn how each of us can choose an enteral nutrition formula that is right for us.

# ❖ 6 ❖

# But My Doctor Says
# It's Not Crohns

## Enteral Nutrition in Ulcerative Colitis, Indeterminate Colitis, and IBS

*They had me on the operating table all day. They looked at my stomach, my gallbladder, they examined everything inside me. Know what they decided? I need glasses.*

**Joe E. Lewis**

We've learned that enteral nutrition can help people with Crohn's. But what if you don't have Crohn's, or aren't sure if you do? This is the chapter for you. In it we will explore the following questions:

• Can people with ulcerative colitis use enteral nutrition?

• Does indeterminate colitis respond to enteral nutrition?

• Does enteral nutrition improve symptoms of irritable bowel syndrome (IBS)?

• Is it okay to use enteral nutrition if you have GI symptoms but no diagnosis?

• Is enteral nutrition safe for people with celiac disease?

Read on to discover the answers.

# What is ulcerative colitis?

**Ulcerative colitis**, like Crohn's disease, is a form of **inflammatory bowel disease** (**IBD**). It is similar to Crohn's in many ways. Both diseases cause inflammation in the gastrointestinal tract, and both can also cause **extraintestinal** symptoms (symptoms that occur elsewhere in the body, such as joint pain and eye or skin involvement).

But there are also differences between ulcerative colitis and Crohn's.

- Inflammation affects the inner lining of the intestine (the **intestinal mucosa**) in ulcerative colitis. It can affect the full thickness of the intestinal wall in Crohn's.

- Intestinal inflammation in ulcerative colitis is limited to the large intestine. In Crohn's, it can affect any part of the gastrointestinal tract from the mouth to the anus.

- Fistulas, abscesses, and strictures are typical of Crohn's, but not of ulcerative colitis.

There are some other differences between the two diseases, but those three are the most important.

# Enteral nutrition in ulcerative colitis

Early studies of enteral nutrition in IBD included people with ulcerative colitis as well as those with Crohn's. Patients with both diseases gained weight and strength from the therapy.[264] Occasionally a person with ulcerative colitis even responded dramatically to enteral nutrition and went into complete remission.[265]

But researchers soon discovered that enteral nutrition does not reduce inflammation and induce remission in people with ulcerative colitis the way it does for those with Crohn's.[266] The rare good responders among those with ulcerative colitis almost certainly had unrecognized Crohn's instead.

❖ **Enteral nutrition is not an alternative to drugs or surgery for people with ulcerative colitis.**

That said, there are times when ulcerative colitis patients can benefit from enteral nutrition—above all, when they are so sick that they are losing weight. Anywhere from one-fifth to two-thirds of people with ulcerative colitis experience at least occasional weight loss.[267] In addition, around 15% of kids with ulcerative colitis have growth delays, often due to malnutrition.[268]

Sometimes people with ulcerative colitis feel too sick to eat. Others aren't willing to eat very much because whatever they do eat runs right right through them. But weight loss and nutritional deficiencies make it much harder to recover from any illness, ulcerative colitis included. Malnutrition also makes surgery riskier.

Enteral nutrition can help provide a balanced diet when you are not up to eating much regular food. If you're only nibbling a little toast and applesauce, an enteral nutrition formula can supply extra nutrients and calories.

There's another advantage, too. Because enteral nutrition products are low-residue liquids, you may produce less stool after drinking them than after consuming the same amount of calories from solid food. When you are fighting severe diarrhea, fewer bowel movements can be a very good thing.

Although doctors once thought that total enteral nutrition would worsen diarrhea or wouldn't be well absorbed by patients with ulcerative colitis, we now know that it is just as well tolerated as TPN in most people with colitis, even those who are seriously ill.[269] It also carries fewer risks of serious complications such as blood clots and infection than TPN.[270]

# Enteral nutrition in indeterminate colitis

**Indeterminate colitis** is the term used to label cases of IBD that are not clearly diagnosable as Crohn's or ulcerative colitis. (It can be very difficult to tell the difference between the two diseases when symptoms of IBD are limited to the colon.) Some people with indeterminate colitis are ultimately diagnosed with ulcerative colitis or Crohn's. Others never fall distinctly into either category.

In one small study, nine patients with indeterminate colitis were treated with enteral nutrition for six to eight weeks. All had significantly improved scores on a colitis symptom score after treatment. Although only three of the participants had biopsies, those that were performed showed reduced colonic inflammation after treatment.[271]

Although it's unlikely that the majority of patients with indeterminate colitis would achieve results as good as these, if you have a diagnosis of indeterminate colitis, you might want to experiment with enteral nutrition for week or two (with your doctor's approval!) to see if you notice any improvement.

A trial of enteral nutrition may also be useful option for patients diagnosed with ulcerative colitis who have noticed symptoms that seem more typical of Crohn's.

❖ **In a recent study, the most common characteristics in patients whose diagnosis changed from ulcerative colitis to Crohn's were weight loss and non-bloody diarrhea at the time of the initial diagnosis of colitis.**[272]

An excellent response to total enteral nutrition—rapid disappearance of symptoms and normalized blood work—is a strong indicator that you may be dealing with Crohn's. But remember that you could still have Crohn's disease even if you don't respond to enteral nutrition.

Enteral nutrition isn't effective for every patient with Crohn's, especially those with disease limited to the large intestine.

### Julie's Story

Tracy's daughter Julie was diagnosed with ulcerative colitis when she was only 20 months old. Now three, her disease no longer responds to steroids, and she's been unable to reach therapeutic levels of azathiaprine. She's been using a semi-elemental formula, Vital Jr., because of severe malnutrition and anemia. She takes it through a nasogastric (NG) tube as a supplement to her regular diet. Tracy says:

"Her diagnosis is ulcerative colitis, but her 'ulcerative colitis' has responded amazingly to supplementary semi-elemental. She's been on Vital Jr. for four months now, and with the exception of a short breakthrough flare, she's been doing wonderfully. One thing I love about what we're doing with the NG feeds is that Julie has great color and looks so healthy! She's even getting a little pudgy . . . beyond the bloating she has from prednisone. She's got a glow and isn't pasty anymore (she's very fair, but even so, you can tell when she's very anemic!). She has energy and she feels great almost all the time. On Christmas Eve we were at Whole Foods buying something I forgot and she was running around the store like a total TERROR! And I've never been so glad to have one of my kids act up! I am so grateful we were allowed to try it because I honestly don't know what would have happened without it!"

# What is IBS?

**Irritable bowel syndrome**, or **IBS** for short, is is what doctors call a diagnosis of exclusion. There isn't a test that tells you for sure if you have IBS. Instead, it's a diagnosis that's made after every other condition with similar symptoms has been excluded. If you've gone through a complete workup—blood tests, a colonoscopy, an endoscopy—and nothing has turned up that meets the criteria of another digestive disease, the diagnosis that remains is IBS.

People who suffer from IBS have symptoms that suggest poor gastrointestinal functioning, such as constipation, diarrhea, pain, and/or bloating. However, doctors can't see any physical changes in the gastrointestinal tract that could be causing the symptoms.

In contrast, the disease process that causes digestive symptoms in people with IBD can be identified through endoscopic examinations and biopsies that reveal damage to the intestines. There is almost always other measurable evidence as well, such as fever or weight loss, or blood tests revealing inflammation or nutritional deficiencies.

## Can I use enteral nutrition to treat IBS?

It's okay to use enteral nutrition if you have IBS. Enteral nutrition is simply food in liquid form, not a drug. In fact, if you are experiencing pain or diarrhea from IBS, you may feel better if you limit your diet to liquids temporarily. With enteral nutrition, you can still get the nutrients and calories you need without eating solid food. Just make sure that you are drinking enough enteral nutrition to supply your complete dietary needs! (Check with your doctor first if you plan to use enteral nutrition for more than a day or two.)

However, enteral nutrition won't cure IBS. Although it reduces inflammation and improves absorption of nutrients in people with Crohn's, IBS symptoms aren't caused by inflammation or malabsorption.

## But do I really have IBS?

If your IBS symptoms are recurrent and severe, you may have wondered from time to time whether IBS is really the correct diagnosis, or whether you might have Crohn's or ulcerative colitis instead.

That is a perfectly reasonable concern. Crohn's in particular can be an unusually difficult disease to diagnose. It rarely affects the entire gastrointestinal tract at once. Instead, it may appear in only one or two places, disappear after a while, and then reappear somewhere else. Complicating matters further, some people with Crohn's have dramatically abnormal blood work, but others display only minor abnormalities, even if they are seriously ill.

Symptoms vary quite a bit, too. One person may have severe weight loss and bloody diarrhea, while another only has nagging abdominal pain and a low-grade fever from time to time.

Many people experience digestive difficulties long before they receive an IBD diagnosis. In one study the average participant had gastrointestinal symptoms for over seven years before being diagnosed with Crohn's.[273] Another group of researchers found that, on average, people with IBD first experienced digestive symptoms 11 years before their IBD diagnosis. The time between the first symptoms and an IBD diagnosis was 48 years for one patient![274]

So if you have IBS, there is always the possibility that your diagnosis could one day change to IBD. This is more likely to happen if you sometimes have symptoms that are not typical of IBS—weight loss or recurrent fevers, for instance—even though you've never quite met the diagnostic criteria for ulcerative colitis or Crohn's.

If you or your doctor have suspected Crohn's in the past, and you are currently suffering from severe digestive symptoms, you might consider asking your physician whether it might be worth trying a course of total enteral nutrition. Without a definitive IBD diagnosis, many doctors are unwilling to prescribe steroids or immunomodulating drugs. Enteral nutrition, in contrast, has few side effects, so it can be an appealing option when the diagnosis is uncertain.

Remember, if you *don't* feel better after starting enteral nutrition, that doesn't mean you definitely don't have Crohn's. Some people with Crohn's don't respond to enteral nutrition.

Similarly, if you do feel a lot better after starting enteral nutrition, that doesn't *prove* you have Crohn's. In most cases, your doctor would still need to find endoscopic evidence of the disease to confirm the diagnosis. But you have something that may be even better than a diagnosis: a safe and simple treatment that helps you feel better, regardless of what you and your doctor call your disease.

### Melissa's Story

Melissa has suffered from chronic GI issues for years. "My diagnosis is still in question," she says, "some say Crohn's, some say not Crohn's but aren't sure what it really is. I have a lot of dysmotility—swallowing problems, gastroparesis (slow stomach emptying), chronic constipation, pelvic dyssynergia—and non-specific inflammation in my small bowel (jejunum and ileum)." Melissa controls her symptoms with enteral nutrition, using an elemental formula, Alpha ENF. She explains:

"I find going on exclusive formula helps reduce symptoms when they get so severe I can't eat or sleep. The rest of the time, I use the formula supplementally (with meals) to help with nutrition since I have so many food intolerances, allergies, and sensitivities. My nutrition has improved quite a bit since adding the formula to my diet—I don't get the low albumin or hair loss any more, I don't bruise as easily, and I have been able to gain and maintain weight better (I was severely underweight a year and a half ago, which led me to first try exclusive elemental). I've been on TPN before for a flare-up of the gastroparesis, and so now when I feel the gastroparesis symptoms getting worse again, I immediately switch to exclusive elemental and it seems to stop the flare after about two weeks. . . . The elemental formula has been a blessing."

# A word about celiac disease

**Celiac disease** is an inherited digestive condition. People with celiac disease have an inability to digest gluten, a protein found in most grains, including wheat, rye, barley, and some others. If you have celiac disease and you eat gluten, it can damage tiny finger-like structures called villi that line the small intestine, making it difficult for you to absorb nutrients from food. People with undiagnosed celiac disease can suffer from diarrhea, weight loss, osteoporosis (from failure to absorb calcium properly), nerve damage (from failure to absorb vitamin B12), and other unpleasant symptoms. The treatment for celiac disease is a lifelong gluten-free diet.

If you suspect you might have celiac disease, ask your doctor to perform a group of blood tests called a celiac panel. If any of those blood tests are positive, then you may need to have an **endoscopy**, a procedure in which a doctor uses a tube with a tiny camera at the end to look inside the small intestine and take biopsies. The diagnosis of celiac disease is confirmed if the villi show characteristic changes that are found in people with celiac disease.

❖ **Don't stop eating gluten until the diagnostic tests are completed!**

Blood tests or an endoscopy done while you are on a gluten-free diet will be negative. Even if you definitely have celiac disease, you will only test positive if you are eating gluten at the time the tests are performed.

# Enteral nutrition and celiac disease

Most but not all enteral nutrition formulas are gluten-free, and therefore are safe for people with celiac disease. If you have both

Crohn's and celiac disease (rare, but possible), it's fine to use enteral nutrition to help control the Crohn's as long as you choose a gluten-free formula.

But if you just have celiac disease, there is no need to use enteral nutrition to treat it. Any gluten-free diet is fine for people with celiac disease; you don't need to restrict yourself to a liquid formula.

If you are not sure if you have celiac disease, *don't* begin a course of total enteral nutrition until you have testing to clarify the diagnosis. If you have celiac disease and use a gluten-free formula as your only food, your celiac symptoms will disappear because you are no longer exposed to gluten. But you won't know whether you have celiac disease or a different problem—Crohn's, for instance—that responded to enteral nutrition.

## WHAT HAVE WE LEARNED?

❖ Enteral nutrition isn't a treatment option for people with ulcerative colitis. But ulcerative colitis patients can still use enteral nutrition to maintain good nutrition and a healthy weight if they're not feeling well enough to eat a balanced diet.

❖ A trial of enteral nutrition can be worthwhile for patients with indeterminate colitis and for those with ulcerative colitis who are unsure of their diagnosis. Failure to respond doesn't rule out Crohn's, but a great response raises a strong suspicion of Crohn's.

❖ People with IBS can benefit from enteral nutrition if they have uncomfortable GI symptoms and would feel better using a liquid diet temporarily. Enteral nutrition can also be worth a try for people with gastrointestinal symptoms who are not sure of their diagnosis.

❖ Enteral nutrition is not necessary to treat celiac disease, but any gluten-free enteral nutrition formula is safe for people with celiac disease.

In the next chapter, we will learn about the different types of enteral nutrition, and what to consider in choosing a formula, whenever your diagnosis may be.

## ❖ 7 ❖

# Decisions, Decisions!

## Choosing a Formula

The mind is like the stomach. It is not how much we
put into it that counts, but how much it digests.
**Alfred J. Nock**

There are dozens of enteral nutrition formulas available today. This chapter will help you understand their similarities and differences, and choose the formula that is right for you. We will:

- learn what enteral nutrition is made of
- find out which ingredients people with food allergies should avoid
- discover which formulas are available in the US and elsewhere
- consider how to obtain insurance coverage for enteral nutrition
- examine whether supplements such as fish oil or probiotics make enteral nutrition formulas more effective.

## What's in my formula?

If you look at the label of an enteral nutrition product, you'll find that the ingredient list contains a long string of unpronounceable chemical names. This may be a turnoff if you're used to heeding dietary advice about eating natural, minimally processed foods. But every food we eat, whether an apple fresh from the orchard or a TV dinner, is broken down by our bodies into the chemicals necessary to sustain human life. The big difference between an enteral nutrition formula and the usual food we consume is that the components of the formula have already been reduced to simpler chemical forms so our digestive system doesn't have to do as much work.

## Protein, carbohydrates and fats

Approximately 10% to 15% of the calories in most enteral nutrition formulas come from whole protein or its components (amino acids and/or peptides). These substances supply our body with nitrogen to build new cells and repair damaged tissues.

Another 45% to 90% of the calories in enteral nutrition products come from sugars and starches, the simplest types of carbohydrates. Carbohydrates provide us with the energy we need to function.

The remaining calories in the formula—approximately 1.5% to 45%—come from fat. Fats, like carbohydrates, are a source of energy. Since human beings can get energy from carbohydrates or fats, formulas low in carbohydrates contain greater amounts of fat and those high in carbohydrates contain little fat.

But it's essential that any formula you choose contains at least some fat. Fat cushions our organs, helps keep us warm, supplies backup energy if we haven't eaten in a while, and forms part of the membrane of each of our cells. Without it we can't absorb fat-soluble vitamins such as A, D, E, and K, and we would lack essential fatty acids that our body can't manufacture on its own.

## What else is in there?

Besides carbohydrates, protein, and fat, ingredients present in much smaller quantities include:

- vitamins and minerals (the same vitamins and minerals you would get from a balanced diet)
- preservatives that protect the formula against bacterial or fungal contamination
- emulsifiers that keep fat evenly distributed in the formula
- anti-caking agents that prevent powdered formulas from clumping
- sequestrants that keep fats from spoiling
- natural and/or artificial flavors to improve the taste of the formula
- stabilizers used for thickening, improving texture, and increasing storage life.

Flavoring packets used to improve the taste of some formulas may contain artificial sweeteners such as aspartame or saccharine. Artificial sweeteners make bitter formulas drinkable. Since they have few or no calories, they don't change the calorie count or balance of carbohydrates in the formula.

## What if I'd prefer a sugar-free formula?

It may be a shock to look at the label of your formula and find that one of the main ingredients is sugar or corn syrup. We are used to hearing dietary advice about limiting the amount of sugar we eat. On the whole, it's good advice. Sugary foods often have little nutritional value. They may supply only minimal amounts of protein, vitamins, or minerals. They are frequently high in fat, and consequently high in calories.

But sugar isn't bad in itself. Even people who eat what they consider a "sugar-free" diet—that is, don't add table sugar, honey, molasses, or any other sweeteners to what they eat—still consume sugar.

Sugar is found in fruits, grains, vegetables, and milk. In addition, many foods contain starch that our body breaks down into sugar.

It's just as well that we can't avoid sugar entirely. *Every cell in our body needs a simple sugar called glucose to function.* (Ever had your blood sugar tested? That's a measure of the amount of glucose in your blood.)

In our regular diet, we get carbohydrates from a variety of foods, and our body breaks them down to get the sugar it requires. If we want, we can restrict sugary treats, and stick to natural sources of carbs instead.

But unprocessed foods that supply carbohydrates, such as vegetables or fruits, contain fiber along with their sugars and starches. They have to be processed to separate out the fiber before they can be used in enteral nutrition products. (Most of the formulas used by Crohn's patients are fiber-free so they can be almost completely absorbed by the small intestine, leaving little waste to be processed by the colon.)

During processing:

- sugarcane and sugar beets are broken down into sucrose (our familiar white table sugar)
- cassava root is broken down into tapioca starch
- corn is broken down into cornstarch
- cornstarch is broken down into corn syrup (also called glucose syrup), corn syrup solids, maltodextrins, and dextrins.

Sucrose, tapioca starch, corn starch, corn syrup, corn syrup solids, maltodextrins, dextrins . . . you might find any of these starches or sugars in an enteral nutrition formula. They are there to supply your body with the energy it needs.

Manufacturers choose a specific carbohydrate based on its price and availability, suitable chemical properties (e.g., good solubility in water), and desired sweetness. Maltodextrin, for instance, tastes only mildly sweet, which makes it popular in sports drinks. Corn syrups are available in varying degrees of sweetness, depending on how much glucose they contain. *There is no evidence that one carbohydrate works better than any other in enteral nutrition formulas. Nor is one any healthier than another.*

## Comparing the formulas

We already learned in Chapter 1 that formulas are assigned to three classes—elemental, semi-elemental, and polymeric—on the basis of their protein source.

- Elemental formulas contain amino acids, the most basic ("elemental") building blocks of protein.
- Semi-elemental formulas contain peptides (amino acids linked together into short chains) or a mixture of amino acids and peptides.
- Polymeric formulas contain whole protein (made up of long chains of peptides).

Besides differing in their protein source, the three classes of formulas also vary in their relative proportions of carbohydrates and fat. Elemental formulas tend to have the most carbohydrates, and polymeric formulas the most fat.

None of these differences seem to have much effect on how well the formulas work.

❖ **Studies show that elemental, semi-elemental, and polymeric formulas are *equally effective* in inducing remission, producing weight gain, and improving growth in children and adults with Crohn's.**[275]

Still, we continue to use the terms "elemental," "semi-elemental," and "polymeric" as a convenient way of grouping formulas. Remembering the distinctions between them can be useful. For example, sometimes a person with Crohn's will respond to one type of formula but not to another.[276] If that happens to you, and you know what type of formula you are using, you can look for a formula in a different class. For example, you could switch from an elemental to a polymeric formula, or from a semi-elemental to an elemental one.

## If they all work the same, how do I choose?

Doctors who prescribe enteral nutrition often have one or two formulas that they know well and recommend. If your doctor is familiar with enteral nutrition, the easiest route is to go with whatever formula he or she suggests.

If your doctor doesn't have a preference, there are a number of considerations to keep in mind as you select a formula. You need to find a product that is available in your region. Not every formula is available everywhere in the world.

Cost can also be a big issue. If you don't have insurance coverage and have to pay for your own formula, think about doing some comparison shopping.

Taste is another factor. Flavor and texture vary greatly from one formula to the next. Particularly if you plan to drink the formula rather than use a feeding tube (see Chapter 8 for information about tube feeding), you may want to sample a variety of formulas to find the preparation most palatable to you. Companies that manufacture formulas will sometimes provide free samples.

If you are purchasing formula for a child, check the recommended age range for each formula you consider. Many formulas made for adults are suitable for older children. However, young

---

### Is my formula elemental or semi-elemental?

In the early years of research on enteral nutrition, researchers didn't always distinguish between elemental and semi-elemental formulas. Amino acid-based formulas were referred to as elemental, but so were those that contained peptides, which we would now call semi-elemental. The older usage, which divides enteral nutrition formulas into two broad classes (elemental and polymeric) rather than three (elemental, semi-elemental, and polymeric), has survived to some extent in Europe.

In the US it shows up mainly as a marketing tactic. Some companies seem to think that "elemental" sounds more appealing to consumers than "semi-elemental," so they describe their semi-elemental formulas as "elemental." But if a product contains peptides or hydrolyzed or partially hydrolyzed protein (another way of referring to peptides), instead of, or in addition to, amino acids, it is semi-elemental rather than elemental in the strictest sense of the word.

---

children, and especially infants and babies, have special nutritional requirements. For that reason, companies that make enteral nutrition products often sell pediatric versions of their formulas. Consult with your doctor to make sure that the formula you choose will meet your child's nutritional needs.

If you have dietary restrictions because of a condition such as diabetes or kidney disease, make sure that the components of your chosen formula are compatible with your recommended diet. For instance, if you have high cholesterol levels or a history of cardiovascular disease, you might need to choose a formula that is relatively low in fat. Food allergies may also be a reason to choose one formula over another.

# Is enteral nutrition safe for people with food allergies?

An estimated 2% of adults and 8% of children have food allergies (young children often outgrow their food allergies).[277]

- A **food allergy** is an immunological reaction to a protein found in food.
- The immune system produces antibodies to fight the offending protein.
- Fats and carbohydrates do not cause allergies.

Because the immune system functions throughout the body, allergies to food proteins can produce systemic symptoms. For example, someone having an allergic reaction to a food might start wheezing and coughing, break out in hives, and have digestive symptoms like cramping or diarrhea.

The foods most likely to cause allergies are milk, soy, eggs, peanuts, tree nuts (e.g., walnuts, almonds), shellfish, fish, and wheat.

## Which are the best formula types for people with food allergies?

Since polymeric formulas contain whole protein, they are most likely to be troublesome to people with food allergies.

Semi-elemental formulas include no whole protein, just peptides. Peptides—small molecules that link together to make proteins—are much less prone than whole protein to cause allergic reactions. Many people with food allergies can use semi-elemental formulas, although some with severe allergies cannot.

Elemental formulas are least likely to provoke allergies because they don't contain any whole protein or even peptides. But if you have a food allergy, you do not necessarily have to use an elemental formula. It depends on what you are allergic to, and the severity of the allergy.

## Choosing a formula if you have milk or soy allergies

Most polymeric formulas contain whole milk proteins, and some include whole proteins from both milk and soy.

If a formula contains whole milk protein, some terms that might appear on the label include *milk, milk protein concentrate, casein, acid casein, calcium caseinate, sodium caseinate, potassium caseinate, whey, whey protein isolate, lactalbumin, alpha-lactalbumin,* or *beta-lactoglobulin.*

If a formula contains whole soy protein, some terms that might appear on the label include *soy protein, soy protein isolate,* or *soy protein concentrate.*

Semi-elemental formulas are also likely to contain milk and/or soy proteins, but in hydrolyzed form. **Hydrolyzed protein** is protein that has been broken down into peptides by the addition of water. When milk or soy proteins are hydrolyzed as they are in semi-elemental formulas, they are much less likely to produce an allergic reaction, but the risk is not eliminated totally. If you have a milk or soy allergy, check with your doctor before using any formula containing milk or soy, whether or not the protein is hydrolyzed.

If a formula contains hydrolyzed milk protein, some terms that might appear on the label are *whey peptides, whey protein hydrolysate, hydrolyzed whey protein, casein hydrolysate, lactalbumin hydrolysate, partially hydrolyzed sodium caseinate,* and others.

If a formula contains hydrolysates derived from soy, terms that might appear on the label include *soy protein hydrolysate* and *hydrolyzed soy protein.*

Elemental formulas don't contain any milk or soy protein, or even peptides derived from milk or soy. They are a good choice for people with severe milk or soy allergies.

However, some elemental formulas contain soy lecithin (an emulsifier) and/or soy oil. Soy lecithin and soy oil can contain small amounts of soy protein from the soybean they are extracted from that escapes removal during the manufacturing process. You may need to avoid these two ingredients if you have a soy allergy.

## Peanut, egg, fish, and seafood allergies

People with peanut allergies should watch out for formulas containing peanut oil (also called arachis oil). Most of the peanut protein is removed in extracting the oil, but small amounts can remain.

Those who are allergic to eggs should check for the presence of the emulsifier lecithin, which can be (although rarely is) derived from eggs. Check with the manufacturer of the formula if the source of the lecithin is not specified and you have a severe egg allergy.

People with fish or shellfish allergies should be aware that some manufacturers have begun to add fish oil to enteral nutrition formulas. These oils can contain tiny amounts of the protein of the fish from which they are extracted.

## Wheat allergies

People with wheat allergies will find plenty of enteral nutrition formulas from which to choose. Most of the formulas that have been tested in people with Crohn's are free of gluten and other proteins found in wheat. The carbohydrates in enteral nutrition formulas generally come from corn, sugarcane, sugar beets, or cassava.

Occasionally one or two flavors of a formula will contain gluten, although other flavors are gluten-free. If your formula comes in different flavors, make sure you check the ingredients of each version.

## Rice allergies

Maltodextrin is one of the carbohydrates most frequently used in enteral nutrition. Although almost all of the maltodextrin used in the US comes from corn, it can also be derived from rice or potatoes. If the ingredient list doesn't specify the plant source of the maltodextrin, ask. Rice-based maltodextrins can contain small amounts of rice protein, although most of the protein is removed during processing.

## A caution for those with food allergies

The range of potential food allergies is too wide to provide a comprehensive list of all the ingredients in enteral nutrition formulas that could possibly provoke an allergy. The preceding paragraphs are meant to familiarize you with some of the more common ingredients that can be problematic, but they are no substitute for consultation with your doctor.

> ❖ **If you have food allergies, speak with your physician before choosing an enteral nutrition formula, and check with the formula's manufacturer for the most complete and up-to-date information on its ingredients.**

# Food intolerances and enteral nutrition

Many people are puzzled about the difference between food allergies and food intolerances. Although they can have similar symptoms, they are not the same thing.

- Food allergies involve the immune system.
- Food intolerances involve the digestive system only.

When someone is allergic to a food, their whole body may react to it. Food allergies can be life-threatening. In contrast, a food intolerance may cause a physical reaction—diarrhea or bloating, for example—but not a systemic immunological reaction.

Food intolerances are much more common than food allergies. Plenty of people complain that certain foods make them gassy or constipated, or give them the runs. Food intolerances can be very individual. One person might react to mushrooms, another to cabbage.

## Lactose intolerance

One of the most common food intolerances is **lactose intolerance**. A person who is lactose-intolerant has difficulty digesting **lactose** (milk sugar), the carbohydrate found in milk. This is because his or her body does not make enough **lactase**, the enzyme that breaks down milk sugar into components we can absorb in the small intestine. If not all of the lactose is broken down, the undigested bits travel on to the large intestine where they are fermented by bacteria that live in the colon. Hydrogen and/or methane gas released during this fermentation process can cause bloating, pain, and diarrhea.[278]

Lactose intolerance is different from being allergic to milk.

- People who are allergic to milk can't tolerate milk protein.
- People who are lactose-intolerant have trouble digesting milk sugar.

Lactose intolerance isn't something you need to worry about much when you are choosing an enteral nutrition formula. Most enteral nutrition products used in Crohn's are lactose-free—even those that contain dairy products. They may contain milk protein, but they don't contain milk sugar.

If you are lactose-intolerant, don't worry if the label of your formula says that it contains dairy products, as long as it is also marked "lactose-free" or "clinically nil lactose" or a comparable phrase.

❖ **People who who are lactose-intolerant but not allergic to milk do not have to avoid formulas containing milk protein.**

## Other food intolerances

Because the ingredients in enteral nutrition formulas are carefully chosen to be easily digestible, it's rare for someone to be intolerant of a food product contained in a formula. But occasionally people react with nausea or diarrhea to formulas that contain ingredients they normally eat without difficulty.[279]

In some cases, a severe flare of Crohn's may have caused them to stop producing normal levels of one or more of the enzymes involved in the digestion of carbohydrates. By switching formulas, they may find a preparation made with a carbohydrate that they are better able to digest at the moment.

More commonly, symptoms such as diarrhea or vomiting that occur after starting a formula are not due to intolerance of a particular ingredient. Instead they occur because the formula is highly concentrated.

## What's osmolality and why does it matter?

The concentration of an enteral nutrition formula is referred to as its **osmolality**. Some people have trouble adjusting to highly concentrated formulas (those with a high osmolality).

If a formula is more concentrated than blood and other body fluids, the gastrointestinal tract may pull water into the intestines to dilute it until it matches the concentration of body fluids. That process can cause diarrhea, nausea, and vomiting.

Consuming your formula slowly, especially when you first begin to take it, can help prevent such symptoms. Also, some people need to dilute their formula with extra water during the first day or so, and gradually transition to drinking it at a normal concentration.

If the nausea and vomiting don't go away, switching formulas can be a good move. Try looking for a formula with a lower osmolality, such as a product whose concentration is similar to that of human body fluids, approximately 300 milliosmols per liter.

If a company makes more than one version of a formula, generally the version with the highest calorie count will have the highest osmolality. For example, a product containing 350 calories per 8 ounces of formula is likely to have a higher osmolality than a version of the same product containing 250 calories per 8 ounces.

But osmolality can vary greatly between formulas, so it is hard to offer general guidelines. One formula supplying 250 calories per 8 ounces might have an osmolality of 350, while another supplying the same number of calories but made by a different manufacturer from different ingredients could have an osmolality of 600. You can usually find osmolality of a formula listed on the manufacturer's Web site.

High osmolality is not necessarily a bad thing. Calorie-dense formulas, which often have high osmolalities, make it possible to drink less formula per day but still get the calories you need. Many people have no difficulty tolerating formulas with high osmolality.

## Choosing an enteral nutrition formula when you have short bowel syndrome

Finding an enteral nutrition formula that works for you may be especially challenging if you have short bowel syndrome. One product may work much better than another at reducing drainage from a stoma, for instance, but there's no way to predict in advance which one will be most effective. A single study reported that high- and low-fat polymeric formulas produced significantly smaller stoma outputs than a semi-elemental formula in people with ileostomies and resections of at least 100 cm of small intestine.[280] But with only one randomized study comparing formulas in people with short bowel syndrome, we don't have enough evidence to predict what formula might be best for any one individual. You may need to experiment with multiple formulas to find the product that suits you best.

One man who had had a total **colectomy** (removal of the colon) and extensive resections of his small intestine agreed to test five different formulas. Only a single one was effective for him (a high-fat semi-elemental formula). The other four formulas (three low-fat or no-fat elemental and one low-fat semi-elemental) were useless because they produced so much drainage from his jejunostomy.[281] But the formula that worked for him will not necessarily be the right one for you.

Luckily you'll have plenty of choices if you want to try enteral nutrition. Elemental, semi-elemental, and polymeric formulas have all been reported to improve nutrient absorption, reduce stoma output, and produce weight gain in individuals with short bowel syndrome.[282] So if you have short bowel syndrome and respond poorly to a given formula, keep experimenting until you find a product that works for you.

## What formulas are available?

Thanks to case reports and clinical studies published in reputable medical journals, we know that over 50 different enteral nutrition products have been used to induce or maintain remission in people with Crohn's disease.

Only four are currently available in the US. The formulas and their manufacturers are: Optimental (Abbott Nutrition), Peptamen (Nestlé Nutrition), Vital HN (Abbott Nutrition), and Vivonex T.E.N

(Nestlé Nutrition). Another formula, Ensure (Abbott Nutrition), has been shown to improve growth in kids with Crohn's, but hasn't been tested specifically to see whether it induces remission.

A few other possibilities for those in the US are Vivonex Plus, Neocate Junior, Osmolite 1 Cal, E028 Splash, and Ensure Plus. Vivonex Plus (Nestlé Nutrition) is close in composition to Vivonex HN, a product that was studied in people with Crohn's. Neocate Junior (Nutricia North America) is similar, although not identical, to an Italian version of Neocate used in a published study. Osmolite 1 Cal (Abbott Nutrition) is close in composition to a discontinued formula, Osmolite, that was studied in some patients with Crohn's. E028 Splash (Nutricia North America) is closely related to Elemental 028 Extra (SHS International), a product that has been evaluated in people with Crohn's but is not sold in the US. Ensure Plus (Abbott Nutrition) has been studied in people with Crohn's, but fiber was recently added to its ingredients, so the composition of the formula is no longer exactly the same as that tested in published reports.

Some well documented products that are not currently available in the US but are sold in Europe, Asia, or elsewhere include Elental (Ajinomoto Co.), Elemental 028 (SHS International; differs in composition from Elemental 028 Extra), and Modulen IBD (Nestlé Nutrition).

There are many other enteral nutrition products available that have not been formally studied in people with Crohn's. Companies develop and market formulas for different purposes. A formula may be positioned as a product for people with kidney disease or patients with diabetes or individuals with cancer or congestive heart failure. It may be low in fat or high in protein to suit patients with particular dietary needs. It may be marketed as a meal replacement product or diet shake and sold in drugstores and supermarkets. It may be advertised only to medical professionals and available through medical supply houses.

Just because a product has not been tested to see if it induces remission in people with Crohn's does not mean that it might not work equally well. If it supplies all the nutrients a human being would need in a day when consumed in reasonable quantities (approximately 1,500 to 2,000 calories), it is potentially suitable for those embarking on total enteral nutrition. Check with your doctor or a registered dietitian to make sure.

Be sure to avoid liquid supplements marked "not for use as a meal replacement" or "not for use as sole nutrition." Even if you drank enough of them to supply your full calorie needs for a day, they would not provide you with a balanced diet.

*You will find contact information for major manufacturers of enteral nutrition products in Appendix B.*

## Are there any vegan or vegetarian enteral nutrition formulas?

Many enteral nutrition formulas that have been tested in people with Crohn's disease include milk protein or proteins from both milk and soy. These products may be suitable for vegetarians who consume dairy products (ovo-lacto or lacto-vegetarians).

In theory, formulas that get *all* their protein from soy should work the same as milk-based formulas. But we don't know for sure. So far no published studies have tested whether soy formulas can induce remission in people with Crohn's.

Elemental formulas might seem a good choice for vegans be-cause they don't contain any whole protein, whether from animals or plants. They are based on amino acids. But be aware that some amino acids are extracted from animal protein. Other amino acids are produced from sugars or syrups by fermentation microorgan-isms. The organisms are stimulated by enzymes to manufacture more of the desired amino acid than they would normally do on their own.[283]

# Modular formulas

In rare situations you may need to use a formula that is specially mixed to suit you from individual ("modular") components. A single module might provide protein, carbohydrate, or fat. Modules are combined to produce a nutritionally complete formula. Alternately, one or more modules can be added to a standard formula to increase its content of certain nutrients.

If you turn out to be intolerant to several different formulas, using a formula made from modular components can allow your doctor or dietitian to change one ingredient at a time to determine which is causing the problem.

# Building a better formula

Formulas with a wide range of ingredients, and with widely varying proportions of protein, carbohydrates, and fats, have all been shown to be effective in inducing remission in people with Crohn's. No single formula type seems to be consistently better than another. But can we make a good formula even better by adding special ingredients— fish oil, for instance, or probiotics? Let's see what studies show.

### Does adding fish oil make a difference?

In recent years, researchers have wondered whether omega-3 fatty acids, found in fatty fish and fish oils, might have anti-inflammatory effects in chronic inflammatory diseases like Crohn's. Some manufacturers of enteral nutrition products have already started to add omega-3 fatty acids to some of their formulas. However, there have been only two published studies testing whether the addition of fish oil to enteral nutrition actually makes a difference for people with Crohn's.

Among 10 patients with Crohn's, a semi-elemental formula seemed to work equally well whether it was supplemented with olive oil or fish oil, but there were too few patients to draw any conclusions.[284]

In a study of 84 children and adolescents with Crohn's, a polymeric diet that did not include any special supplementation and a semi-elemental diet enriched with an omega-3 fatty acid were equally effective in inducing remission.[285]

With data from only two studies, it's too early to draw any firm conclusions. But so far there is no evidence that fish oil-supplemented formulas are any more effective than standard enteral nutrition products at inducing or maintaining remission in Crohn's disease.

## Should I look for a glutamine-enriched formula?

Glutamine is an amino acid that helps protect the intestinal mucosa. For that reason, researchers wondered if increasing the amount of glutamine in enteral nutrition formulas might make them more effective. But a randomized study showed that a polymeric formula enriched with extra glutamine wasn't any more effective at getting children with Crohn's into remission than a similar formula containing normal amounts of glutamine.[286]

The take-home message: there is no need to choose a formula with extra glutamine in it.

## Should I choose a formula containing a probiotic?

**Probiotics** are microorganisms that may be beneficial to their hosts and are nonpathogenic, meaning that they do not normally cause disease. They are often advertised to health-conscious consumers as supplements that can help improve intestinal health.

As yet, there has not been a single published study testing whether enteral nutrition formulas with probiotics in them can induce remission in people with Crohn's, or whether formulas with and without probiotics differ in their ability to induce or maintain remission. So at least for now, there is no reason to look for a formula containing a probiotic.

## Should I look for a formula containing a prebiotic or other type of fiber?

In spite of advertising touting their benefits for digestive health, **prebiotics** are nothing more then some common types of fiber gussied up with a fancy name. Typically prebiotics contain two types of fiber, inulin and oligofructose, that are also referred to as fructooligosaccharides, or FOS for short. They occur naturally in thousands of plant species, including many that make part of the normal human diet. Because prebiotics aren't absorbed by the body, they are often used to add fiber to foods without adding calories.[287]

Although consumption of fiber is often seen as valuable to good intestinal health, we don't know yet whether adding a prebiotic to an enteral nutrition formula makes that formula more, less, or equally effective in inducing or maintaining remission.

So far, only one fiber-containing formula has been tested in a published study of patients with Crohn's. The study included 84 children, and half of the kids received a formula that included prebiotics (fructooligosaccharides).[288] Those who received the formula with prebiotics had a 62% remission rate, so the fiber doesn't seem to have had adverse effects. However, there wasn't a comparison group of children using a fiber-free version of the same formula, so we still don't know for sure whether adding prebiotics improves, worsens, or doesn't affect a given formula's effectiveness.

Based on the evidence currently available, there is no reason to avoid formulas containing prebiotics, but also no reason to favor them over fiber-free formulas.

# Do-it-yourself enteral nutrition?

A doctor pointed out over 25 years ago that no study of patients with Crohn's had ever compared an enteral nutrition formula with a normal diet puréed into liquid in a blender.[289] Could it be that what matters is consuming a liquid diet, not the exact composition of the liquids? We don't know for sure. But we do know that some people with Crohn's feel better if they temporarily limit their diet to liquids, even without using special enteral nutrition formulas.

One gastroenterologist routinely recommends a one- or two-day-per-week liquid diet to his patients with small intestinal Crohn's who develop abdominal pain or obstructive symptoms while waiting for their maintenance medications to take effect. (If the two-day-per-week schedule is chosen, each liquid diet day is separated by two or three days eating thoroughly chewed normal food.) The patients are allowed to use any food that can be made into a liquid, as well as any beverage, including enteral nutrition formulas.[290]

If you try this tactic, make sure to choose liquids that will provide your full daily nutritional requirements! Juices and clear soups are not enough. Weight loss and malnutrition can be very dangerous, especially during a flare of Crohn's.

The big advantage of using a prepared formula is that you know it will include sufficient calories, along with all the nutrients you need in a day—protein, fat, carbohydrates, vitamins, and minerals.

### Jen's Story

"Basically, when I start to flare I go on mostly liquids for a few days. I don't use any official formulas. I just buy smoothies when I'm out and about or I will make one with Slim-Fast powder, protein powder, bannana, yogurt, ice, and soy milk. I also drink Pedialyte to keep my electrolytes up. I figured this out on my own so that I was strong enough to continue working as a corrections officer without spending my whole shift in the bathroom. From there I start to add in bland foods . . . applesauce, banannas, bread, yogurt (more or less the BRAT diet). Then I move on to plain chicken, etc., until I'm back to normal. If I catch it early, I just do the liquids for a day or two. I know I have avoided a lot of flares and steroids this way."

# Where can I buy enteral nutrition?

Some enteral nutrition products, such as Ensure or Boost, are sold in drugstores and grocery stores in the US. Other formulas have to be ordered from the manufacturer or through a pharmacy or medical supply house. Contact the manufacturer for suggestions if you are unable to find a local source of supply.

Be sure to order the correct version of your formula. Some formulas are available in two different versions, one designed for tube feeding, the other for drinking. Formulas made for tube feeding are unflavored, and most are undrinkable (or at least extremely bitter!). If you plan to drink your formula from a glass, look for a version that has flavoring added, or that can be made palatable by adding flavor packets.

## Can I purchase it without a prescription?

Generally, yes. In the US, most enteral nutrition formulas are classified as medical foods or dietary supplements, which do not require a prescription, rather than as drugs, which do. However, since medical foods are meant to be used under a doctor's supervision, some manufacturers may ask you for a doctor's order before making the sale.

## What is the difference between a prescription drug, a medical food, and a dietary supplement?

Prescription drugs are intended to prevent, treat, or cure diseases. They cannot be sold in the US unless they have been tested first to determine whether they are safe for human use and whether they do what they are intended to do. Before the FDA approves a drug, it assesses the studies performed by the manufacturer and determines whether the claims made about the product are valid.

In contrast, dietary supplements do not have to go through a testing process and be approved by the FDA before they are placed on the market. Because they do not have to undergo the same level of scientific scrutiny as prescription drugs, the companies that make them are not allowed to claim that dietary supplements can prevent, treat, or cure disease.

Medical foods fall in a middle ground between prescription drugs and dietary supplements. Like dietary supplements, they do not have to go through a testing and approvals process before being placed on the market, and manufacturers of medical foods cannot say that their products prevent, treat, or cure disease. But medical foods have to meet certain requirements that dietary supplements do not.

To be classed as a medical food in the US, a product must be:

- suitable for oral or tube feeding
- intended for use under medical supervision
- specially made for the dietary management of a specific medical disease or condition that has distinctive nutritional requirements.

The ingredients of medical foods must be listed completely on their labels, beginning with the ingredient present in the largest amount and ending with that present in the smallest amount.

❖ **Medical foods such as enteral nutrition formulas were originally regulated as drugs by the FDA. In 1972 the agency reclassified them to encourage their wider development and availability.**

In some countries—Japan, for instance—at least some of the enteral nutrition formulas used in Crohn's disease are regulated as drugs rather than as medical foods or nutritional supplements.

## Does it matter whether my formula is a medical food or a dietary supplement?

If you are going to use a product to supply all your dietary needs, it's good to know exactly what's in it. Makers of nutritional supplements are under no obligation to provide a complete ingredient list to consumers, and many do not. That makes it hard to tell if you're getting sufficient quantities of all the vitamins and minerals you need. In contrast, complete labeling is a requirement for manufacturers of medical foods.

That said, medical foods are not necessarily superior to dietary supplements. If a supplement company provides clear and complete labeling, and adheres to reputable marketing and production standards, its product may be just as reliable as a medical food.

It's not always clear from a manufacturer's advertising whether a given formula is a dietary supplement or medical food. Clues to medical food status are a statement that the product is designed to be used under medical supervision and the presence of a detailed ingredient list, but the only way to determine the status for sure is to ask.

## Obtaining insurance coverage for enteral nutrition

*Note: The following paragraphs are aimed primarily at readers in the United States. However, they may be relevant to those living elsewhere who are struggling with insurance issues related to enteral nutrition use.*

Most of the time US health insurance companies pay partially or in full for prescription drugs. Sometimes for financial or other reasons they will limit their policyholders' choice to certain medications in a given class—for example, not covering a branded drug if a generic option is available—but generally if you have health insurance and your doctor prescribes a medication, you will not have to pay the whole price yourself.

The situation can be very different if you need enteral nutrition. The formulas used for enteral nutrition are typically classed as medical foods or nutritional supplements rather than prescription drugs. As a result insurance companies treat them as they would over-the-counter medications: as nonessential products that consumers use by choice and should pay for themselves. Insurers may also argue that their policies cover medications and medical services, not food.

But don't give up if you receive an initial denial. You may be able to win coverage using your company's appeals process. The key factor is that enteral nutrition is not just any type of food. When used in people with Crohn's, it is a special form of nutrition used to treat a specific illness. It produces clinically significant improvement that can be verified with blood tests and disease activity indices. It acts like a prescription drug, even though it is a nonprescription food. Consequently, even if an insurance company refuses to cover enteral nutrition initially, it may reverse its position after you make your case.

Usually you will need to obtain a letter from your doctor supporting the therapy and supply documentation showing that it is a medically validated treatment (one that has been proven effective in clinical studies published in reputable medical journals). The information in this book should provide plenty of ammunition for your battle. Alternately, you may find it easier to give your insurance company a copy of this book.

If you do end up paying for your own enteral nutrition, some or all of the cost of the formula, if it is prescribed by your doctor to treat a specific medical condition, may be deductible on Schedule

A of your federal tax return (if you itemize your taxes rather than claiming the standard deduction). See the Internal Revenue Service's Publication 502, Medical and Dental Expenses, for more details and be sure to check with your tax advisor about whether this deduction applies to your particular situation.

## Do you live in Massachusetts, New York, or New Hampshire?

If you live in one of those three states, obtaining coverage for total enteral nutrition is likely to be much easier for you than for those living elsewhere in the United States. Laws in all three states require insurance companies to cover the cost of enteral nutrition formulas for gastrointestinal diseases such as Crohn's when the prescribing physician (or in New York, any licensed health-care provider legally authorized to prescribe) has written a letter stating that the formula is medically necessary.

- In New Hampshire, refer your insurance company to New Hampshire Insurance Statutes, Section 415:6-c.
- In New York, cite New York Insurance Law, Sections 4303[y], 3216[i][21], and 3221[k][11].
- In Massachusetts, the relevant statutes are General Laws of Massachusetts, Part I, Title XXII, Chapter 176A, Section 8L; Chapter 176B, Section 4K; and Title IV, Chapter 32A, Section 17A.

In New Hampshire, nonprescription enteral nutrition formulas are covered "for the treatment of impaired absorption of nutrients caused by disorders affecting the absorptive surface, functional length, or motility of the gastrointestinal tract." A doctor's written order needs to affirm that the formula "is needed to sustain life" and "is the least restrictive and most cost-effective means for meeting the needs of the patient."

In New York, besides indicating that the enteral formula "is clearly medically necessary," the doctor's order must state the formula "has been proven effective as a disease-specific treatment regimen" for the patient's health problem. The statute specifies that enteral nutrition formulas have been proven effective for the following conditions: "inherited diseases of amino acid organic acid metabolism; Crohn's disease; gastroesophageal reflux with failure to thrive; disorders of gastrointestinal motility such as chronic intestinal pseudo-obstruction; and multiple, severe food allergies which if left untreated will cause malnourishment, chronic physical disability, mental retardation, or death."

In Massachusetts, enteral nutrition formulas are covered for home use when a physician has issued a written order and the formula is "medically necessary for the treatment of malabsorption caused by Crohn's disease, ulcerative colitis, gastroesophageal reflux, gastrointestinal motility, chronic intestinal pseudo-obstruction, and inherited diseases of amino acids and organic acids."

It's not clear whether coverage for supplemental enteral nutrition would be required under these laws. Total enteral nutrition is clearly a treatment for a disease, whereas enteral nutrition supplements could be seen in some cases simply as nutritional support. However, someone who has life-threatening weight loss if he or she does not continue to supplement with enteral nutrition could conceivably fall under the New Hampshire criteria of requiring the formula "to sustain life."

In New York, the relevant statutes include a clause indicating that "enteral formulas which are medically necessary and taken on the written order from a physician for the treatment of specific diseases shall be distinguished from nutritional supplements taken electively." Potentially a supplement essential to keeping someone in remission and properly nourished might be classed as medically necessary rather than elective.

The Massachusetts criteria seem most inclusive, as the formula needs only to be medically necessary for the treatment of malabsorption. That would seem to apply to supplemental enteral nutrition for those who develop nutritional deficits without it.

Wherever you live, the first thing is to make a convincing case for enteral nutrition to your insurer. Then you may have to wait and see how the situation plays out.

## WHAT HAVE WE LEARNED?

❖ In people with Crohn's disease, elemental, semi-elemental, and polymeric formulas are equally effective. There is no evidence that formulas supplemented with fish oil, glutamine, probiotics, or prebiotics work better than unsupplemented formulas.

❖ Enteral nutrition formulas are considered medical foods or nutritional supplements, not prescription drugs. You do not need a doctor's prescription to purchase enteral nutrition, but your insurance company may require you to have a prescription for it in order for the company to cover the cost of the formula. If your insurance company refuses to pay for enteral nutrition, you may be able to win coverage on appeal.

❖ Issues to consider in choosing a formula include taste, cost, availability, physician preference, special dietary needs, and food allergies. People with lactose intolerance can use formulas that contain milk protein but are lactose-free.

Now that we've learned about choosing a formula, in Chapter 8 we will find out how to successfully start—and complete—a course of enteral nutrition.

## ❖ 8 ❖

# Go For It!

## Using Enteral Nutrition

> Changing our diet is something we choose to
> do, not something we are forced to do. Instead
> of dreading it, I try saying, "Here's another
> thing I get to do to help myself. Great!"
> **Greg Anderson**

If you've decided to try enteral nutrition, this chapter is for you. Here's where you'll find the answers to practical questions you might have before, during, or after treatment. You'll learn:

- how to talk with your doctor about using enteral nutrition
- whether you need to take medications or supplements along with it
- whether it's better to drink the formula or take it through a tube
- how to figure out how much formula you need
- whether you might experience any side effects from enteral nutrition
- how long you should continue using enteral nutrition
- how to reintroduce regular food after completing enteral nutrition.

# Convincing the doctor:
# why use enteral nutrition?

Your doctor might not have treated many patients with enteral nutrition or might not have prescribed it at all. He or she may ask why you would choose this treatment over other options. If you've read this far, you probably know your reasons already. But here are some possibilities: to avoid the side effects of corticosteroids, to regain lost weight, to improve growth (for children), because the medications you've tried didn't work or no longer work, because you are worried about the possibility of drug-related side effects, because you want to postpone using immunomodulating or biologic drugs as long as possible, because you can't afford biologic drugs and you've tried everything else without success, or because you would prefer a nutritional rather than a drug-based approach to treatment. Make sure your doctor knows you are willing to consider using medication if enteral nutrition doesn't work!

If your doctor is still uncomfortable prescribing enteral nutrition, ask why. Someone who is seriously malnourished and acutely ill may need aggressive care, using every available treatment, to avoid a potentially life-threatening crisis. If your doctor has reservations about using enteral nutrition, listen carefully. Enteral nutrition is a great treatment for *some* people, *some* of the time; it is not always the right treatment for every person and every situation.

❖ **This book is not a substitute for a doctor's education, training, and experience.**

But if your doctor's reservations about enteral nutrition are mainly because he or she isn't very familiar with it and assumes that it doesn't work or is rarely effective, perhaps you might suggest a short trial period. You could agree to have blood tests to assess inflammation a week or two after starting enteral nutrition, and indicate your willingness to consider switching to another therapy or adding a medication to the mix if you have not begun to improve in that time period.

### Jerry's Story

Alice's teenage son Jerry, who has ileal and rectal Crohn's disease, was treated with prednisone after his initial diagnosis. When he relapsed a few months later, he agreed to try enteral nutrition instead. "He was really, really motivated to try it because he hated his experience with prednisone," Alice says.

Jerry's doctors at a big US children's hospital were surprised at his choice. Alice describes her conversation with one of them:

"When I told her Jerry was in a flare, I explained I had learned of a liquid diet option from another mom whom I'd met on the Internet. She was silent on the phone for a few long seconds, at which time I said, 'This is okay, isn't it?' She replied by saying something like, 'Oh yes, but we have never had anyone actually do it.' She then went on to confirm that studies support it as effective as prednisone to stop a flare. Overall, she seemed quite amazed that Jerry was undertaking this liquid diet, but didn't discourage me from allowing it."

Jerry responded quickly to total enteral nutrition, and was able to begin reintroducing solid foods to his diet after only nine days of treatment.

## What if my doctor wants me to use TPN instead?

Ask your doctor why he or she wants you to use TPN. Is it simply that the doctor is more familiar with and more comfortable with TPN? Or is there a special reason why TPN is best in your case? As we learned in Chapter 1, six different studies have compared TPN with enteral nutrition in people with Crohn's, and every one of these studies found that TPN and total enteral nutrition (whether with elemental, semi-elemental, or polymeric formulas) were *equally effective* in producing remission.[291] Enteral nutrition has the additional benefit of being less expensive and causing fewer complications.[292]

Although serious complications of TPN are rare, they do occur. Among a hundred patients with Crohn's disease who used TPN on a long-term basis, four died of complications directly related to the use of TPN.[293] Another group of 41 Crohn's patients who were long-term TPN users included three people whose deaths were caused by complications of TPN.[294]

The purpose of mentioning these studies is not to scare you away from *appropriate* use of TPN. Sometimes enteral nutrition is *not* a suitable treatment—if you have a complete bowel obstruction, for instance, or your intestines have stopped working entirely. In these situations, TPN is absolutely essential, and its benefits far outweigh the small risk of complications. Remember, the vast majority of people who use parenteral nutrition do so without problems or with only minor difficulties, and need it for only a short period of time. But why take any risk if you don't have to? As long as your intestines are functioning at least partially, total enteral nutrition works just as well as TPN, without the safety worries of parenteral nutrition.[295]

## Do I need to take steroids along with total enteral nutrition?

Total enteral nutrition can be used on its own. Most studies have found that patients improve just as quickly on enteral nutrition as on steroids.[296] Weight gain, too, is equally good.[297] Using a steroid and total enteral nutrition at the same time is no more effective at improving weight and nutritional status than using enteral nutrition alone.[298]

Using a steroid simultaneously can make it harder to comply with enteral nutrition because of the food cravings that accompany steroid use. However, if you are already taking a steroid when you start total enteral nutrition, *never* discontinue it abruptly! Steroids need to be tapered slowly. You can do that during your first weeks on enteral nutrition.

The one compelling reason to *start* steroids when you are on enteral nutrition is if you've been complying with the diet for a week or so without response, and your health is getting worse. In that case, it's very important to start another therapy without delay.

## Can I use immunomodulating medications at the same time as enteral nutrition?

If you are already using immunomodulating medications such as 6-MP, azathioprine, or methotrexate, it is fine to continue them while you are using enteral nutrition. They will not change the effectiveness of the nutritional treatment. Since immunomodulators can take several months to become effective, some people start one at the same time that they begin enteral nutrition. The nutritional treatment gives them a way of controlling painful symptoms during the weeks before the drug therapy takes effect.

## Can I take metronidazole or aminosalicylates during enteral nutrition?

If you have perianal disease or fistulas, you may already be taking metronidazole (Flagyl), or your doctor may have suggested that you start it. It's fine to take metronidazole when you are using total enteral nutrition. Doing so can be a good idea because perianal disease and fistulas can be very difficult to treat nutritionally, even in people whose other gastrointestinal symptoms heal quickly on a liquid diet.

If you are already taking an aminosalicylate (sulfasalazine or a mesalamine drug such as Pentasa or Asacol), you may continue it during enteral nutrition use. However, if you are not taking a medication in this class currently, you may want to avoid starting one at the same time as enteral nutrition. Since aminosalicylates can cause diarrhea in some people, it can be difficult to tell whether you are responding poorly to an enteral nutrition formula or having a bad reaction to the drug.

## In a cup or through a tube?

If you decide to use enteral nutrition, your next decision will be how to take it. You can drink enteral nutrition from a glass like any other beverage or take it through a tube that delivers the formula directly to your stomach or small intestine.

❖ **It doesn't matter how you consume your chosen formula. However it gets to your gastrointestinal tract, it works exactly the same.**

Let's look at the options.

### The simplest approach: just drink it

Drinking the formula has some big advantages: there are no tubes to insert, no special equipment to maintain. No one needs to know that you are on a special diet. With the popularity of meal replacement drinks and sport beverages, you probably won't stand out if you are drinking your lunch at work or at school, especially if you carry the product in a reusable water bottle or thermos. Challenges you may face include getting used to the taste of the formula, managing to drink enough each day to meet your nutritional needs, and adjusting psychologically to not being able to eat your favorite foods temporarily.

To get you started on the right foot, here are 10 tips for success:

1. Consider drinking your formula at regular meal and snack times together with others who are eating so you are not deprived of the social pleasures of meals.

2. If you're heading out for the day, take an extra serving or two of formula with you. Cheating on the diet becomes much more tempting if you don't have formula available when you're hungry.

3. If you can't stand the flavor, don't give up without giving your taste buds a chance to adjust. Within as little as three days most people adapt and no longer find the taste of their diet unpleasant.[299] If your formula comes in different flavors, sticking to the same flavor can help you adjust to the taste more quickly.

4. Experiment with the temperature of the formula. Many people think that enteral nutrition formulas taste best chilled, but others prefer them at room temperature.

5. If you find the smell of the formula unpleasant, put the liquid in a covered container and drink it through a straw.

6. If you feel nauseated or bloated after drinking your formula, try consuming it more slowly. Some people do better if they sip a portion slowly over the course of half an hour rather than chugging it down all at once.

7. Brush your tongue regularly while using enteral nutrition. Otherwise the formula can build up on your tongue, forming a coating that tastes and feels unpleasant.

8. Regular tooth brushing after each liquid "meal" helps to prevent cavities.

9. Enjoy the fact that your food preparation and clean up is now so simple: nothing but opening a bottle or mixing a powdered

formula with water. Use the time you've saved to give yourself a treat—go to a concert or sports event, for instance.

10. If you are tempted to quit, make a list of the reasons you decided to try enteral nutrition in the first place (e.g., getting to remission, avoiding medication side effects, etc.). Focus on those benefits. Are they important enough that you could put up with enteral nutrition for just one more day? Would your life really be that much different if you could eat whatever you wanted right now as opposed to waiting a few weeks for the treat? Take it one day at a time, and keep reminding yourself of the upside of the treatment.

## Would tube feeding be a better option?

Drinking the formula is not for everyone. You might want use a tube instead if you:

- have ulcerations in your mouth or throat that make swallowing uncomfortable
- have persistent nausea or vomiting when you try and drink your formula and consuming it more slowly doesn't help
- can't tolerate the taste of any of the formulas you've tried
- can't drink enough of the formula to meet your calorie requirements
- prefer to get all your nutrition during the night rather than drinking the formula during the day.

A feeding tube is also a good choice for very young children who need enteral nutrition. Many older children successfully drink the enteral nutrition they need, although others prefer a tube or must be switched to tube feeding because they are not willing to comply with a liquid diet.

### Bill's Story

Bill was diagnosed with severe Crohn's at the age of two. He was treated with antibiotics, steroids, an immunomodulating drug, a 5-ASA drug, and supplemental enteral nutrition given through a nasogastric (NG) tube. His doctors even considered starting Remicade. His condition stabilized, but he continued to have active disease after the steroids and antibiotics were withdrawn. His mom, Gail says:

"Because Bill always looked better on enteral nutrition, we started to think about it as a longer-term strategy for him. Fortunately, at the time Bill was going to an excellent day-care facility, and the day-care director approached me about the possibility of teaching him to drink the formula. We had been told that the formula was bad-tasting and perhaps undrinkable, which was a particular problem for our son who was the pickiest eater on the planet. However, the day-care director and a counselor we were seeing at the time helped us work through the logistics of getting Bill to drink the formula. We put flavor packets in the formula, and had Bill drink it at special times like bath time when he would associate the drink with happy events. We even got a bowl of little bouncing balls and other prizes that he could take after he drank it. Although we started with just sips of formula at a time, he later drank small cups of it, and within some number of weeks was drinking about two cans a day reliably. For the next five years he drank the formula and has never had to go back to an NG tube."

## Nasogastric, nasoduodenal, and nasojejunal tubes

There are different types of feeding tubes. The most common, the **nasogastric tube**, is inserted through the nose and ends in the stomach (from *naso* = nose + *gastric* = pertaining to the stomach).

Patients—even children—can learn to put in their own nasogastric tube. Some kids and adults insert one at night, and then remove it in the morning so no one can see they are using a tube to eat. Other people find inserting and removing the tube uncomfortable. They leave it in place until they are done with their enteral nutrition regimen.

Less common are **nasoduodenal tubes** (inserted through the nose and ending in the duodenum) and **nasojejunal tubes** (inserted through the nose and ending in the jejunum). These tubes bypass the stomach, delivering the food directly to the small intestine. (The **duodenum** and **jejunum** are the first and second sections of the small intestine.) Nasoduodenal and nasojejunal tubes may be a good choice for people with severe gastroesophageal reflux (regurgitation of stomach acid) that causes nausea and/or vomiting. The disadvantage is that you can't take these tubes in and out yourself the way you can with the nasogastric variety.

❖ **If you need to leave a tube in place, some people may notice it and stare. But it's your attitude that counts, not theirs. You can't control what they do, but you can choose whether to allow it to annoy or upset you.**

There are relatively few complications to worry about with nasogastric tubes or other tubes inserted through the nose. Probably the most annoying is the discomfort associated with the insertion of the tube and the feeling of having it there in your nose. Although some people find these sensations intolerable, most get used to the presence of the tube quickly and find they are able to ignore it. Occasionally a tube becomes dislodged accidentally (during sports, for example, or at night), but with practice and a little tape, you will become adept at keeping it in place. There is a small risk of inserting a tube into the wrong place (such as the lung) or perforating the esophagus, but such serious complications are very rare.

### Daniel's Story

Daniel has been using enteral nutrition supplements for about five years, with occasional courses of total enteral nutrition (learn more of his story in Chapter 5). His mother Sharon says:

"You can lead a totally normal life whilst using this treatment—my son inserts an NG tube each night for overnight feeds and removes it in the morning. To all intents and purposes he is a perfectly normal 18-year-old, he studies full-time and has a part-time job as a lifeguard, does several sports, and is off to university in September. He is nearly six foot and weighs about 68 kilograms [150 pounds]. Our first-ever doctor told us his prognosis was poor, he had ulcers the full length of his gut, and he would never make a good adult height. What a difference five years makes!"

## Gastrostomy tubes

Not all children and adults are comfortable with tubes inserted through the nose. They find them uncomfortable to insert and remove, or are embarrassed if they have to leave a tube in place where others can see it. Another choice is hooking up the tube to a **gastrostomy**, a small, artificially created opening that leads from the outside of the body into the stomach. This is a good option if you or your child needs enteral nutrition on a long-term basis. Compared with a nasogastric tube, there are no daily worries about getting the tube in the right place, dislodging it accidentally, or looking different from everyone else. (The gastrostomy site is hidden by normal clothing.)

If you choose this option, you aren't stuck with a gastrostomy permanently. Once you are back to normal diet and no longer need the gastrostomy tube, the tube is removed. The opening that remains is closed with a minor surgical procedure if it doesn't heal up on its own.

The disadvantage of a gastrostomy is the need to create the artificial opening used for feeding. Typically this is done in one of two ways. In a surgical gastrostomy, a small slit is made externally in the abdomen and a tube passed through it into the stomach. In a percutaneous endoscopic gastrostomy (PEG), a tube is inserted through the nose and passed down to the stomach. Its end is brought out to the surface of the abdomen through a small incision made in the skin from the interior, using an endoscope to determine the placement of the opening.

Whichever technique is used, complications are generally minor: leakage around the mouth of the gastrostomy tube; skin irritation from the leakage; local infection or buildup of inflamed tissue around the gastrostomy site. Sometimes the original tube wears out and has to be replaced, or a longer tube must be substituted because of growth or weight gain. Very rarely, a gastrostomy tube leaks internally, or a fistula from the stomach to the skin develops after the tube is removed, rather than normal healing.[300]

## Getting the formula into the tube

No matter what type of feeding tube is used, the formula is pushed or dripped into the tube from a syringe or bag several times a day (**bolus feeding**) or dripped continuously through the tube by a pump (**continuous-drip feeding**).

Bolus feedings mimic how human beings normally eat: with most food consumed during three meals per day, and sometimes a couple of snacks as well. But if you can't tolerate large amounts of formula all at once, or can't get enough nutrition in several feedings per day, continuous-drip feeding can be a big help.

You can hook up the pump in the evening and get the formula overnight or use it continuously throughout the day. Those who have to consume the formula at a very slow rate to avoid nausea may keep the pump running day and night to get as much nutrition as possible. Backpacks are available (including some designed for children) so you can carry the pump with you.

## How do I prepare the formula?

Some formulas come ready prepared in bottles or cans. All you have to do is open the container and drink, or empty the contents into a clean feeding bag if you are tube feeding. Other formulas are supplied in powdered form and have to be mixed with water before use. If you are drinking the formula by mouth, you may have to add a flavor packet before consuming it.

Whatever type of formula you are preparing, make sure to wash your hands before you start, whether you are mixing formula for yourself or someone else. Once you have opened a bottle of formula or mixed powdered formula with water, keep the product refrigerated if you are not going to use it right away. Discard any formula you haven't used within 24 hours.

If you are tube feeding overnight or for a number of hours at a time, make sure the formula is cold when you start to slow bacterial growth. The feeding bag shouldn't be hung at room temperature for more than 8 to 12 hours. Check the instructions for your particular product.

Nutrients may start to degrade after the formula is opened or mixed. In at least one case, the vitamin C content of a formula dropped dramatically when it was stored overnight after preparing it, even when the product was refrigerated.[301] Of course, it's not always possible to prepare formula right before consuming it, particularly if you have to bring it with you to school or work. Simply try, whenever possible, to prepare it as close to the time you need it as you can.

# How much formula do I need if I want to try total enteral nutrition?

Generally you will drink the same amount of calories that you would eat if you were consuming solid food. For instance, if you typically need 1,800 calories per day to maintain your weight on a normal diet, then you will likely need about 1,800 calories per day of formula. But calorie requirements vary from person to person, and you may have to experiment to find your ideal level of consumption, particularly if your activity level varies from day to day. If you are in the middle of a flare, you may need more calories than the normal recommended daily allowances for your age and gender to maintain your current weight, and an even higher calorie count to gain weight.[302]

Once you've calculated the amount of calories you need, check the nutritional data for the formula you have chosen and make sure that you will be consuming enough of the formula to get at least the minimum daily requirements of each vitamin and mineral.

For growing children using total enteral nutrition, the usual rule is to determine the child's ideal weight (rather than actual weight!) for his or her age, and provide the amount of calories that would be needed to maintain that ideal weight.[303]

Those whose weight is normal or who are overweight do not have to put on extra pounds to benefit from enteral nutrition.[304] Enteral nutrition reduces intestinal inflammation and improves nutrient absorption even without increased calorie consumption. If you don't need weight gain, your doctor or dietitian can help you to figure out the amount of enteral nutrition you will need on a daily basis to maintain your weight rather than increasing it.

If you have drunk your appropriate calorie allotment for a meal and still feel hungry, try drinking a glass of water to remove the sweet taste of the formula from your mouth. Then leave the table and busy yourself with something else for 15 minutes or so. Once the stimulating taste of sugar in your mouth is removed and your stomach has time to realize it's full, you will probably realize you don't need more to eat.

## If I'm supplementing my regular diet with enteral nutrition, how much formula should I use?

The amount of supplement you need depends on your goal: gaining weight, maintaining remission, or, for children, improving growth. It may take a few days to figure out the balance between formula and regular food that is right for you.

Approximately 500 to 600 calories of enteral nutrition per day can help you gain weight and reverse nutritional deficiencies. That usually works out to about two cups.

Upping the amount of formula to 750 calories or more per day can help maintain remission, as we learned in Chapter 4. If your weight is normal when you begin supplementing, you may need to reduce the amount of regular food you eat to avoid gaining weight from the addition of the supplement.

What about for kids? Studies have shown excellent growth in children who supplement their diet with 1,000 or more calories of enteral nutrition per day (some teenagers use up to 1,800 calories).[305] Other children may do fine with smaller amounts. For instance, an 11-year-old girl started growing again once she began using 500 calories per day of enteral nutrition.[306] (See Chapter 3 for more details about supplemental enteral nutrition for children.)

It doesn't matter whether your child prefers to drink the formula during the day or take it through a tube overnight, the supplement works just the same. You may need to decrease the quantities of enteral nutrition and/or regular food you feed your child once he or she reaches a normal weight. Growth does not require excessive weight, only normal weight proportionate to height.

## Do I need to take any dietary supplements along with my enteral nutrition?

Enteral nutrition formulas are designed to provide all the nutrients you need. If you are using total enteral nutrition, generally you won't have to take any additional vitamins or minerals unless your doctor recommends them to make up for particularly severe deficiencies.

## Can I have anything except the formula?

If you are using enteral nutrition supplements, you'll be taking them alongside your normal diet. But the rules are different if you are starting total enteral nutrition. Typically people using total enteral nutrition are asked not to eat or drink anything besides the formula except water.

But some doctors permit patients to drink tea or coffee without milk during enteral nutrition use as well.[307] Lollipops, similar hard candy, and sugarless gum are often allowed, too, and can make it easier to cope with not having anything to chew on.

If you are using any prescription medications, you should continue to take them while utilizing enteral nutrition unless your doctor advises you otherwise.

## Will the formula interact with any medications I am taking?

There have been very few interactions reported between prescription or over-the-counter drugs and enteral nutrition formulas. Those interactions that are known are described below. But if you take any medication or supplements, it's safest not to mix them into your enteral nutrition formula. Although interactions rarely occur, they are not impossible. When you dissolve one substance in another, you never know what chemical reaction you might produce (think about how yeast bubbles up in warm water and sugar or the way baking powder fizzes if you add it to vinegar).

## Warfarin (Coumadin)

The anticoagulant warfarin (also sold under the brand name Coumadin) may be less effective if you are using enteral nutrition due to an interaction with vitamin K contained in enteral nutrition formulas. Your doctor should monitor your warfarin levels if you begin treatment with enteral nutrition. Usually any problems can be solved by switching to a formula with less vitamin K.[308]

## Phenytoin (Dilantin)

The epilepsy drug phenytoin (also sold under the brand name Dilantin) may not reach effective levels in the blood if it is given at the same time as an enteral nutrition formula. That means that you won't be properly protected from seizures. If you take phenytoin, check with your doctor before starting enteral nutrition and see what he or she recommends. A common approach is to not take any enteral nutrition from at least two hours before until at least two hours after a dose of phenytoin. If you're using a feeding tube to take both your enteral nutrition formula and phenytoin, be sure to flush it out before and after taking the medication.[309]

## Antacids

If aluminum-containing antacids are given through the same tube as an enteral nutrition formula, they can cause the formula to thicken, potentially obstructing the esophagus. If you need to take antacids while using a feeding tube, make sure to wait for a while after a feeding and then flush the tube first before using the antacids. Never add aluminum-containing antacids directly to a formula.[310]

There are many varieties of aluminum-containing antacids (for example, Basaljel, Amphojel, Alu-Tab, Maalox, Mylanta, Graviscon, etc.), so check with your doctor if you take an antacid and aren't sure what type it is.

### Potassium

If you take an oral potassium preparation, don't mix it into your enteral nutrition formula if you are taking the formula through a tube unless you've checked with your doctor first. The mixture may coagulate and cause the tube to clog.[311]

### Iron

Mixing an iron supplement into an enteral nutrition formula may drastically decrease the amount of vitamin C in the feed. Instead take the supplement separately.[312]

# Does enteral nutrition cause any side effects?

Most people adapt easily to enteral nutrition formulas with few or no problems.

❖ **There is no reason to fear a trial of total enteral nutrition. Remember this isn't medication, it's nothing but food, simply food in liquid rather than solid form.**

If you have any complications at all, they will almost always be minor. Here are some of the issues that you might (but probably won't!) need to manage.

## Nausea or bloating

Some people develop some nausea or bloating, or even a little mild abdominal pain, during the first few days after they begin to use total enteral nutrition. (Admittedly, if these are typical Crohn's symptoms for you, it may be difficult to tell what's Crohn's and what's side effect. But don't worry unless you experience anything that's markedly different from your usual pattern.)

These minor gastrointestinal symptoms usually go away quickly. Try sipping the formula more slowly over a longer period of time (if you are drinking it) or slowing the rate of administration (if you are tube feeding). It may also help to temporarily reduce the amount of the diet you are consuming and then slowly increasing the quantity, or diluting the formula and increasing it gradually to full strength over several days.

(To learn more about why these side effects may occur, see the section of Chapter 7 titled "**What's osmolality and why does it matter?**")

## Constipation

It's hard to believe, but you can become constipated on an all-liquid diet, even if you don't normally experience anything except diarrhea. If constipation occurs, try drinking at least two or three glasses of water a day in addition to your enteral nutrition. That will usually reverse the problem (of course, talk to your doctor if it doesn't). Even though enteral nutrition preparations are liquids, many people need more fluids than they get from the formula.

## Diarrhea

One of the big advantages of total enteral nutrition is that Crohn's-related diarrhea often clears up speedily. But sometimes people develop diarrhea after starting total enteral nutrition, usually from consuming the formula too rapidly or because it is too concentrated for them to tolerate easily. As with nausea or bloating, diluting the formula or slowing down your rate of drinking or tube feeding can solve this problem quickly.

But severe diarrhea, sometimes accompanied by vomiting, that starts after beginning total enteral nutrition can also be a sign that you are intolerant of the formula. (See the section on food intolerances in Chapter 7 for more details.) If you develop severe diarrhea after starting total enteral nutrition and it does not improve within two or three days even if you slow down your rate of consumption, don't try and stick it out. Just switch formulas.

It's usually best to try a distinctly different type of formula. For instance, if you started with a very low-fat elemental formula, switch to a higher-fat polymeric one. If you were using a polymeric formula, switch to an elemental or semi-elemental one. In addition, try and find a formula that's made with a different type of carbohydrate or different mix of carbohydrates than the one with which you started.

## Allergic reactions

If you are allergic to milk or soy, you may have to choose your formula carefully to avoid exposure to these ingredients, as described in Chapter 7. But with these exceptions, it is exceedingly rare for ingredients in enteral nutrition formulas to provoke allergic reactions. In a single reported case, a patient developed a rash caused by either the flavoring agent or dye in a raspberry-flavored version of an elemental formula.[313] If you do develop a rash or other allergic-type reaction after starting enteral nutrition, by all means report it to your doctor immediately. But don't worry too much about this! The risk for such a complication is extremely low.

## Headaches and/or dizziness

If you are on total enteral nutrition, and go for a long time without consuming any formula, you may develop a headache or feel sweaty or shaky. This can be a sign that your blood sugar has become low (hypoglycemia). If you are prone to hypoglycemia, try drinking small quantities of formula more frequently. Make sure that you are getting enough water, too, because dehydration can cause dizziness or faintness.

## Refeeding syndrome

One rare but potentially serious complication that could occur during the use of enteral nutrition is **refeeding syndrome**. This is a disturbance in the body's balance of fluids and **electrolytes** that can occur when people who are malnourished begin to receive proper nutrition.

Refeeding syndrome is not a problem that occurs only with enteral nutrition. It can happen whenever malnourished patients gain weight, whether with solid food, enteral nutrition, or TPN.[314]

---

### What are electrolytes?

Electrolytes are substances, mainly minerals, that have positive or negative electric charges when they dissolve in body fluids or water. The electric charges affect the movement of fluids and nutrients in and out of cells.

Electrolytes help regulate muscle contractions, heart rhythm, blood clotting, conduction of nerve impulses, and other bodily functions. Important electrolytes include sodium, potassium, phosphate, calcium, chloride, magnesium, sulfate, and bicarbonate.

---

Paresthesias (pins and needles sensations) in your hands and feet and muscle weakness are the two of the most common early warning signs of refeeding syndrome.[315] *If you notice these, or other disturbing symptoms, seek medical care immediately.* A doctor should check your electrolyte levels as soon as possible and adjust them as necessary. You may also need to temporarily reduce the quantity and concentration of the formula you are taking, but this is not an adjustment you should make on your own. Left untreated, refeeding syndrome can cause delirium, seizures, bone pain, liver damage, cardiac complications, and even death.[316]

But don't let these potential complications scare you away from enteral nutrition. Doctors have been treating Crohn's disease with enteral nutrition for some 40 years. In that time there have been only two confirmed published cases of refeeding syndrome in Crohn's patients using enteral nutrition, and two additional possible cases.[317] It probably occurs more frequently than this—not all complications of any medical treatment are published in medical journals—but it is certainly not an everyday occurrence. Mild, transient disturbances of fluids and electrolytes that resolve on their own are much more common. Even if you do experience refeeding syndrome, that doesn't mean you have to discontinue enteral nutrition or that it's not going to work for you. But you will need prompt medical care to reverse the problem so you can continue treatment safely.

## Rhabdomyolysis

A very few people using an elemental diet for Crohn's disease have developed rhabdomyolysis, a condition in which muscle cells break down and release a substance called myoglobin that can damage the kidneys.[318] Doctors are not 100% sure why this happens, but the occasional patient with long-standing malnutrition may not be able to tolerate the large amounts of carbohydrate found in some formulas.[319] Reducing the amount of formula taken per day reverses the problem, but this should be done under a doctor's supervision.

Muscle weakness is the most common easily recognizable symptom of rhabdomyolysis. *If you notice muscle weakness after starting treatment with enteral nutrition, call your doctor immediately.* Refeeding syndrome is the most likely explanation for this particular symptom, but if you have muscle weakness in spite of normal electrolyte levels, make sure to have your creatine phosphokinase level checked. Levels of this enzyme rise when rhabdomyolysis occurs.

### Essential fatty acid deficiency

In a handful of cases, essential fatty acid deficiencies have been reported in people using total enteral nutrition.[320] The formulas they used didn't supply the minimum daily requirement of linoleic acid or alpha-linolenic acid, two essential fatty acids.

With modern enteral nutrition formulas, you are highly unlikely to develop a fatty acid deficiency from enteral nutrition. But see your doctor if you begin to notice skin abnormalities during enteral nutrition use, especially if you are using a very low-fat formula (such as a product with less than 5% of calories from fat). Dermatological symptoms such as skin atrophy or dermatitis (an itchy, red rash) are often the first visible sign of essential fatty acid deficiencies.

## Getting started: the first day

There are several ways to start total enteral nutrition. Beginning all at once is appealing to many people. You can set a "D-Day" to get started, plan a last meal in advance with all your favorite foods, and be off and running with your new treatment the next day. But starting with normal quantities of full-strength formula is not always a wise move. It can increase the possibility of suffering a little nausea or bloating or diarrhea during the first day or two, and raises the risk of refeeding syndrome. Check with your doctor first to make sure you don't need a more gradual approach. But some patients can start directly on full-strength formula without difficulty.[321]

Alternately, you might prefer to ease into total enteral nutrition by adding a little bit more of your chosen formula to your diet every day until by the third or fourth day you are getting all your nutrition from it and have discontinued solid food entirely. This gradual approach can help you adjust to the taste of the diet and get used to consuming large amounts of liquid. The disadvantage can be that if you're all psyched up to start total enteral nutrition, you might lose some of your momentum and enthusiasm during those first few days. It may also take you a little longer to benefit from total enteral nutrition, since you won't be fully on enteral nutrition until several days after starting.

Another option is to switch directly to total enteral nutrition without tapering solid food, but dilute the formula with extra water at the beginning and slowly increase the concentration or drink less than the recommended amount of formula during the first day or two and work up to the full amount. This approach can help prevent gastrointestinal side effects such as bloating or diarrhea. Accompanied by careful monitoring of fluids and electrolytes, it can be the safest way to start total enteral nutrition for people who have a higher than normal risk of refeeding syndrome, such as those who are elderly, severely malnourished, or have a history of cardiovascular or kidney disease. The downside of beginning with a decreased concentration or quantity of formula is that you might lose a little weight in the first day or two, or suffer some headaches or dizziness.

❖ **Talk to your doctor about which approach to starting total enteral nutrition is right for you.**

# Will I still have bowel movements since the diet is all-liquid?

Yes, but they may be less frequent than you're used to, especially after you've been using the formula for a while. On average, healthy volunteers who participated in a ten-day test of enteral nutrition formulas had one bowel movement every one and a half to two and a half days.[322] In a nineteen-week study, some healthy people using total enteral nutrition had bowel movements as infrequently as once every seven days.[323]

Your stools may be liquid, and they may look greenish also, when you are using total enteral nutrition.

# When will I know if enteral nutrition is going to work?

You will probably begin to feel considerably better within ten days, even if you are not in full remission that soon. In fact, many patients are lucky enough to see noticeable improvement within the first two or three days.

❖ **In a large series of patients with Crohn's, symptoms improved within one week of starting the diet in 90% of attempts at total enteral nutrition that ended in full remission.**[324]

Unfortunately, if you haven't seen any improvement at all in two weeks, and none of your labs look better, enteral nutrition may not be the treatment that works for you.[325] However, the occasional patient will respond if given a little extra time, and may start to show improvement closer to the three-week mark.[326] Also, sometimes a patient who tolerates but does not respond to one enteral nutrition formula does respond if switched to another.[327] (Likewise, some patients who respond to one enteral nutrition formula will relapse if switched to a different one.[328])

Just how long you continue with enteral nutrition if you're not responding is up to you. It can be terribly frustrating to get your hopes up about a treatment, comply with it conscientiously, and then have no results. But it is the unfortunate truth that total enteral nutrition, like every other treatment for Crohn's, is not effective for everyone. All you can do is try it and see.

## How long should I stick with enteral nutrition?

The amount of time for which people use enteral nutrition varies greatly. In one survey, gastroenterologists reported treating patients with total enteral nutrition for anywhere from five days to 16 weeks.[329] We don't know if there is an ideal duration of treatment that will maximize the length of remission.[330]

In all events, it makes sense to continue treatment until your symptoms are gone and your blood work is normal. Continuing for least a week or two after you reach that stage *may* help consolidate your gains, but no one really knows.

If you are using supplemental enteral nutrition as a maintenance treatment, it can be continued indefinitely. Sticking with it can reduce your risk of a relapse.

## How soon will my child start growing after beginning enteral nutrition?

Expect improvement in weight to come before increased height. When someone is malnourished, the body's first priority is to replenish needed stores of vitamins, nutrients, and fat. Only then does it have extra resources to devote to growth.

But once your child has put on some weight, he or she is likely to benefit from several months or more of rapid growth, even after discontinuing enteral nutrition.

## What will happen if I cheat on the diet?

When you are using total enteral nutrition, the ideal is not to eat or drink anything except the formula. Both kids and adults can find this a considerable challenge. Among teenagers tube feeding with total enteral nutrition, one of 14 who responded to a questionnaire and four of 11 interviewed in person acknowledged sometimes sneaking foods in secret. Grown-ups may not be much more compliant. In a series of adults treated with total enteral nutrition, over 20% of the patients confessed that they ate normal food occasionally, at least one did so frequently, and a few others cheated once.[331]

It's hard to say just how much cheating you can do (if any) without affecting your chances of reaching remission. But we know that people who use total enteral nutrition are considerably more likely to reach remission than those who consume a mix of enteral nutrition and regular food.[332] If you can stick with the liquid formula and avoid eating any other food, you will have the best chances of success.

*If you do break down and cheat on the diet, don't decide you've blown it and give up.* Just accept the mistake and go back to total enteral nutrition. It's not very different from being on a weight loss diet and splurging on a pint of ice cream. Yes, it would be better if you hadn't done it, but getting up the next morning and resuming the diet is far more productive than quitting because of one mistake.

It may help to make a list of at least five or six activities that you could do to distract yourself if you find yourself craving food. Activities that take you out of the way of temptation, such as a walk around the block, may be particularly useful. But keeping yourself busy with almost anything can help. Once you are engaged in another pursuit, you are likely to forget about the food craving or find that it subsides enough to be manageable.

## Is it cruel to make a child stick with enteral nutrition?

Parents have a wide range of attitudes toward enteral nutrition. Some think it would be terrible for their child and for the whole family. Others are convinced that it is the best possible option.

The treatments available to your son or daughter at a given moment are likely to influence your decision. Enteral nutrition is not an easy choice. But uncontrolled Crohn's isn't pleasant either, and nor are the side effects of some of the medications used to treat it.

Selecting this particular treatment for Crohn's is a decision that has to seem right to your family. The story below describes one family's decision-making process.

### Matthew's Story

Matthew was diagnosed with ulcerative colitis at the age of six. "Scopes showed that he had open sores dripping blood from end to end of his large intestine," says his mother, Gail. (Matthew's brother Bill also has IBD, and his story appears earlier in this chapter.)

A couple of years later Matthew's diagnosis changed to Crohn's. "We tried all kinds of medications to bring him into remission," Gail says. "He was already on Asacol [mesalamine] and Purinethol [6-MP], but we added fish oil, probiotics, guided imagery, metronidizole, and Entocort [budesonide]. When we added six cans a day of enteral nutrition a day but still let him have food, his symptoms disappeared but his labs continued to worsen."

"Giving up on enteral nutrition, we introduced even higher-dose steroids for many months, but Matthew still was not getting better. Our doctor felt that the biologic infusions were necessary and we went to a doctor at an IBD center who agreed. Still, my husband and I were uncomfortable about the possible side effects of the biologics."

Gail and her husband discussed the issue. "We couldn't imagine Matthew not eating. He loved food! In fact, when the GI asked Matthew some months back if he thought he could do an exclusive elemental diet for eight weeks, Matthew clearly said, 'No.' Yet while I thought we couldn't do it, I was also wishing that we could. My husband and I went out to dinner, outlined all our options, and made a decision that felt like the right choice for us—we would try enteral nutrition before we put another medication in Matthew's body. I think having talked everything through, both believing this was the best choice for him at the time, and making a formal commitment to it made a huge difference. I also think we took ownership of this decision as parents. We care a lot about our son, and about what he wants, but just as a family wouldn't let the kids decide any number of major issues (for example, whether they'll take medications or not). We felt this really was a parental decision. We made a doctor's appointment to make sure we really had to do something more. When our doctor said we had a choice of another scope so he could show us why Matthew needed Remicade, or we could start enteral nutrition, we sat down and really talked with our son. He hates scopes! So he agreed in theory that enteral nutrition would be better."

Matthew began using an enteral nutrition formula, Peptamen Junior. Within 2 ½ weeks, his symptoms were gone, his ESR (a marker of inflammation) had dropped from the 60s to single digits, and all of his other labs were improving. Gail says:

"My son even said to us, 'Why didn't you have me do this sooner?' I will tell you why, before we did it, who knew! I will say that the no-food part was very difficult for him, and sometimes for us. We went to a few holiday parties but declined many more.

Sometimes he felt so sad that he couldn't eat the birthday cup-
cakes brought to his classroom. When we reintroduced foods, I
did a lot of shopping and cooking! But we will all say, Matthew
included, that this was one of the best decisions we ever made.
He developed a sense that he could control his own disease, and
when he's encountered problems, he himself has chosen to use
this method of resolving them. So far, every time he has, his medical problems have gone away. Also, he's developed a great sense
of self-esteem. Talk about taking on a difficult challenge and really
meeting it head on! And as a reward for one round of total enteral
nutrition, he earned a puppy, who is definitely the light of his life.
So many good things have flowed to him from this decision."

## What is the best way to reintroduce solid food?

When your doctor clears you to return to a normal diet, the temptation is to eat a big meal with all your favorite foods immediately.
Although some people do all right with that approach, it can be
risky. When you have been drinking liquids for a while and sud-
denly consume large amounts of solid foods, you can become nauseated easily or develop stomach pain or vomiting.[333] It's safer to
introduce increasing amounts of solid food at each meal, together
with decreasing amounts of enteral nutrition, for the first day or
two. Occasionally people prefer to go even more slowly, introducing a normal diet over the course of four or five days.

Others prefer to reintroduce foods individually or in small groups
over a period of several weeks or more, to try to identify items that
might trigger a flare. But such food-testing protocols tend to identify
few if any problematic foods. When 29 children received one new
food every two days after completing a course of total enteral nutrition, none identified any problematic foods.[334] Food groups were
reintroduced at weekly intervals in another group of children, and

no specific food group produced symptoms.[335] When food intolerances do occur, they tend to be transitory, with the problem foods causing no symptoms when reintroduced on another occasion.[336]

For most people, it's probably unnecessary to go through a food-testing process. But we'll take a closer look at food-testing regimens and food-exclusion diets in Chapter 9.

## I'm gaining too much weight since I finished using total enteral nutrition. Why?

After patients with Crohn's disease go into remission, they sometimes begin gaining more weight than they'd like. If you have been suffering from active disease and malabsorption for a long time, you might be used to consuming more than the normal caloric requirements for someone your size to avoid becoming skeletally thin. But once your disease is in remission and you have normal absorption, you may have to adjust your intake.

## If enteral nutrition works for me, how long will I stay in remission?

Unfortunately, there aren't any guarantees. Some people are unlucky enough to relapse within a few days of resuming normal food. Other individuals benefit from a year or more of remission after a single course of total enteral nutrition.

One study looked at 53 children who were given total enteral nutrition as their initial treatment for Crohn's disease. A total of 34 (64%) reached remission, and they stayed in remission anywhere from 2.7 to 305 weeks—quite a range! The median length of remission was 21.4 weeks (approximately five months).[337]

In a study of adults, eight of 17 who responded to four weeks of treatment were still in remission six months after the end of the study.[338] In another study, six of eight adults who responded to two weeks of treatment were still in remission 12 months later; the other two relapsed within eight months.[339]

Even very long courses of enteral nutrition will not necessarily extend remission more than shorter courses once the nutritional treatment is discontinued. It seems to be more the luck of the draw and the individual course of the disease. A child who received total enteral nutrition for an entire year was still in remission eight years later, while another treated for the same length of time relapsed after 18 months.[340]

## It's been less than a month since I finished a course of enteral nutrition and I've already relapsed. What should I do?

If you only stuck with total enteral nutrition for two or three weeks, and weren't completely symptom-free when you discontinued the diet, it may be worth trying again for longer. However, if you were in full remission for at least a week or two before you discontinued total enteral nutrition (e.g., no symptoms, normal labs), and yet still relapsed in under a month, then you may need a maintenance treatment to keep you in remission. You could try supplemental enteral nutrition or consider a maintenance medication such as an immunomodulator.

### Carolyn's Story

Carolyn chose enteral nutrition as her initial treatment after being diagnosed with Crohn's in the ileum. She writes:

"My diagnosis of Crohn's disease came as a surprise. I did not feel 'sick enough' to have Crohn's at the time of my diagnosis, and to be honest, I still do not. My main complaints were brief episodes of fever and moderate abdominal pain. I was suffering mild abdominal cramping daily, but my bowel movements were normal and I was not losing weight. However…my gastroenterologist felt I was at risk for severe disease and recommended I immediately begin steriods and azathioprine."

Carolyn was worried about the potential side effects of the drugs, especially since she was still recovering from a liver injury caused by another medication. "Being a student I had access to medical journals, so I searched for alternatives and found enteral nutrition. It seemed like a safer way to remission. I brought printouts of recent medical journal articles to discuss with my doctor, to formulate a course of action for my treatment. However, he would not even consider enteral nutrition. He said it did not work and felt that my decision to try exclusive enteral nutrition was equivalent to 'doing nothing' to treat my Crohn's. He was obviously not pleased that I was choosing enteral nutrition over his recommendation, but he did give me a referral to see a nutritionist after I asked for it."

With the help of a nutritionist, Carolyn chose a polymeric formula, Nutren 1.5 Fiber. She transitioned to total enteral nutrition over the course of a week, replacing one meal per day with a can of the formula. Initially, the formula made her queasy, but she diluted it with water and that helped, as did the rapid improvement. "Luckily after only a few days—while still transitioning—my abdominal cramps lessened significantly," Carolyn reports. She remained on total enteral nutrition for eight weeks, switching to a fiber-free version of the same formula, which she found more palatable, after the first three weeks. Her C-reactive protein and ESR (markers of inflammation) went down into the normal range for the first time in a year, and her doctor declared her in remission. She developed mild elevations of two liver enzymes during treatment, but these normalized after she switched to supplemental enteral nutrition to maintain remission (two cans of formula per day supplemented by small meals and snacks).

Unfortunately, Carolyn began to relapse only three weeks after switching from total to supplemental use of the formula. "This is essentially where my story ends," Carolyn says. "I am still trying to find my way with enteral nutrition, now taking more calories per day from formula versus food, and I am also incorporating additional supplements such as probiotics, omega-3 fatty acids, and vitamin E. I am hoping that I can find a compromise between formula and food that will keep me in remission but still allow some freedom. If that is not possible then I will eventually incorporate medications into my treatment program."

## If I use enteral nutrition, will I be healthier in the long term?

In Japan, total enteral nutrition or TPN have been the standard first-choice treatments for patients hospitalized with Crohn's disease since the 1980s. Immunomodulating drugs such as 6-MP and azathioprine were rarely prescribed until recently. Yet a long-term follow-up study of Japanese patients found that their clinical courses, operation rates, and long-term survival were similar to those that have been reported for patients with Crohn's in Western countries where nutritional treatments are rarely used and immunomodulating drugs are prescribed frequently.[341] This suggests that there is more than one possible way to treat Crohn's.

Yet observational studies such as this don't allow us to draw any firm conclusions. We don't have any randomized, head-to-head studies that compare how people do on a long-term basis when they treat their Crohn's disease with enteral nutrition when it is first diagnosed, and perhaps return to enteral nutrition to deal with relapses, as opposed to beginning treatment with steroids, immunosuppressants, or biologic drugs such as Remicade. What will happen 20 years down the line to a child who begins treatment with total enteral nutrition compared with a child who starts a biologic right after diagnosis?

How will their current health compare? How well will they have done over the years? For now, we just don't know.

## WHAT HAVE WE LEARNED?

❖ Enteral nutrition can be used alone or alongside other medications. But using a steroid together with enteral nutrition may not be any more effective than using enteral nutrition on its own.

❖ Enteral nutrition works equally well whether you drink it or take it through a tube. For those using total enteral nutrition, it's best not to eat or drink anything except the formula, water, and any prescribed medications. Sucking candies, sugarless gum, and tea or coffee without milk may be okay, too. It's better to take any medications or supplements separately rather than mixing them into the formula.

❖ After completing a course of total enteral nutrition, it's safest to reintroduce foods slowly over one or two days, rather than eating a big meal all at once.

❖ Side effects of enteral nutrition are usually minor. The most common are nausea, bloating, constipation, and diarrhea. Much more rarely people using enteral nutrition can develop an imbalance of electrolytes called refeeding syndrome. Starting enteral nutrition gradually or with a reduced concentration of formula can reduce the risk of refeeding syndrome and other gastrointestinal side effects.

❖ Most people who respond to enteral nutrition begin to see improvement within the first ten days, although occasionally someone doesn't begin to respond until the end of two or three weeks. The length of remission after a single course of total enteral nutrition can vary from a few days to over a year. Supplemental enteral nutrition can extend the length of remission.

In the next chapter, we'll examine whether any supplements or special diets other than enteral nutrition can help keep Crohn's under control.

# ❖ 9 ❖

# Beyond Enteral Nutrition

## The Real Truth About Diet in Crohn's

For my part, I mind my belly very studiously, and
very carefully; for I look upon it, that he who does
not mind his belly, will hardly mind anything else.

**Samuel Johnson**

You're finally in remission. Maybe you've even been taking enteral
nutrition supplements but now you're ready to stop them. So
what next? Will you stay in remission longer if you restrict what you
eat or consume particular foods? Is it better to eat a high-fiber or a
low-fiber diet? Are fish oil supplements or probiotics worth it? You
will find the answers here. This chapter explores what researchers
have discovered in studies of diet in people with Crohn's.

## Fiber or not?

Many patients with Crohn's disease assume that their intestinal disease will be less troublesome if they restrict the amount of fiber
in their diet. But are they right? Researchers in Bristol, England,
decided to test the issue. They instructed the Crohn's patients in
their practice (including those with intestinal strictures) to eat more
fruits and vegetables and less refined sugar, and replace white flour,
white rice, and other refined carbohydrates with whole grains.

After noticing that their patients seemed to be doing unusually
well, they decided to compare them with other Crohn's sufferers in

179

the same city who had not been given any special dietary advice. Over an average follow-up period of 4⅓ years, their own patients were significantly less likely to have been hospitalized and had had significantly shorter hospitalizations. They were also less likely to have had intestinal surgery. Only 1 of their 32 patients had needed surgery (for a problem that was already present before he started the diet), compared with 5 of the 32 comparison patients.[342]

These promising results prompted researchers to plan larger trials to see whether dietary fiber really made a difference in controlling Crohn's. In one study, a group of Italian patients were randomly assigned to follow a low-residue diet or a normal diet for approximately two years. Those assigned to the low-residue diet were told to avoid nuts, legumes, whole grains, and all fruits and vegetables except ripe bananas, skinned potatoes, and pulp-free juices.

Although patients with obvious strictures were excluded, most of the 70 participants had active Crohn's disease on entering the study. Nevertheless, individuals who ate a normal diet without fiber restrictions were no more likely than those following the low-residue diet to require surgery or suffer a severe flare, partial obstruction, or inflammatory mass.[343]

A much larger trial produced similar results. Over 350 patients with inactive or mildly active Crohn's disease were randomly assigned to follow a low-fiber or a high-fiber diet for two years. Those assigned to the low-fiber diet were advised to eat refined carbohydrates such as white flour and white rice, consume as much sugar as they wanted, and avoid unrefined carbohydrates such as whole grain foods. The other patients were told to do exactly the reverse: avoid any foods containing sugar or white flour and eat carbohydrates only in their unrefined state.

Two years later, the results were in. There were *no* significant differences between the two groups: not in the number of patients needing surgery or hospitalization, nor in the proportion who completed the trial without experiencing worsening disease. There were not even any obvious differences in outcome when the analysis was restricted to the patients who had complied most closely with their assigned diet.[344]

## But . . .

Regardless of the results of these studies, there are times when you need to be cautious about fiber consumption. If you've just completed a course of total enteral nutrition, a three-course meal heavy on raw vegetables and whole grains is probably not the best choice for your first dinner of solid foods. As described in Chapter 8, you may want to take it slow for a day or two as you return solid food to your diet.

In addition, if you know you have strictures, especially if you tend to have bouts of partial obstruction, you may need to be very cautious about eating fibrous foods that could become trapped in the narrowed areas.[345] Also, sometimes a flare-up of Crohn's can cause transient symptoms of obstruction because segments of the intestines are inflamed. At those times, too, it can be wise to steer clear of foods that could get stuck, such as nuts, seeds, or fibrous vegetables. Make sure to ask your doctor if you have any question about whether you should eat fibrous foods.

❖ **But most of the time, for most patients with Crohn's disease, there is no reason to restrict dietary fiber.**

## Testing a low-carb diet

Thanks to the prior studies, we can see that replacing refined with unrefined carbohydrates or vice versa doesn't seem to have any particular effect on the course of Crohn's. But what about reducing carbohydrates across the board? Given the current popularity of low-carb diets, you might be wondering how they work for people with Crohn's.

In the only study that looked at this issue, a low-carb diet (<84 grams per day of carbohydrate) didn't provide any special benefit over a normal diet.[346] However, compliance with the low-carb diet was so poor that we can't draw any firm conclusions from the results. But there is no reason to think that a low-carb diet would have any particular value in Crohn's disease. Elemental diets providing 70% or more of their calories as carbohydrate have gotten plenty of people with Crohn's into remission.

## Should I worry about yeast?

Yeast is a popular villain in alternative health circles these days, with many people blaming it for digestive symptoms. People with Crohn's disease tend to produce higher levels of antibodies to a yeast called *Saccharomyces cerevisiae* (more commonly known as baker's yeast) than individuals without IBD. So could reducing yeast consumption reduce Crohn's symptoms?

Unfortunately, things don't seem to be that simple. One small study tested this hypothesis by comparing a normal diet with a low-yeast, low-sugar diet (sugar was restricted in an attempt to limit intestinal yeast growth). While on the low-yeast, low-sugar diet, the patients were instructed not to eat breads, malted cereals, dairy products, alcohol, vinegar, sauces, gravy-browning or stock cubes, vitamin D supplements, mushrooms, sugar, preserves, white flour, fruits, or any foods containing fruit.

These dietary restrictions didn't have any noticeable effects. Disease activity wasn't any different when the patients were on the yeast-free diet than when they were eating their normal diet. Additionally, levels of antibodies to *Saccharomyces cerevisiae* didn't change significantly when the patients were limiting yeast.[347] At least on the basis of this study, reducing consumption of foods con-taining yeast and sugar seems unlikely to make much difference in controlling Crohn's.

## Microparticles aren't the answer

Several studies have examined whether tiny inorganic particles found in Western diets as food additives might set off intestinal inflammation or make it worse. These naturally occurring "microparticles" (the size of bacteria) turn up as colorants or anti-caking agents in products as diverse as salad dressings, toothpaste, snack foods, and sweeteners.[348] We also consume microparticles inadvertently as soil and dust (on unwashed fruit, for example).

A small pilot study suggested that a diet low in microparticles might help Crohn's patients treated with steroids reach remission faster.[349] But two much larger studies found that avoiding micro-particles didn't make any difference. In one, steroid-treated patients randomly assigned to a normal or low microparticle diet were equally likely to reach remission.[350] In the other, there were no significant dif-ferences in microparticle intake between people with Crohn's and healthy volunteers.[351]

The verdict: restricting microparticle consumption is unlikely to be effective in preventing or controlling Crohn's.

## All the fish in the sea

Omega-3 fatty acids found in fatty fish and fish oils have received plenty of good press lately. Researchers are exploring whether diets rich in omega-3 fatty acids might help protect us against conditions as diverse as Alzheimer's disease, depression, and cardiovascular disease. Could the omega-3s also be beneficial in chronic inflam-matory diseases like Crohn's? So far, the evidence is mixed.

Results from a small, randomized study suggested that patients with Crohn's might benefit from regular consumption of fish or fish oil. Over the course of two years, participants instructed to take fish oil supplements or one meal of cold water fish or fish pâté per week had fewer relapses than individuals who were assigned to continue with their normal diet.[352]

Another promising study included 38 children with Crohn's who were treated for a year with a 5-ASA drug plus a fish oil supplement or the same 5-ASA drug plus a placebo. By the end of the year, 61% of the children who received the fish oil had relapsed, but no relapses had occurred until after the eighth month of treatment. In contrast, 95% of those who received the placebo had relapsed, with the first relapses occurring after only 1 month of treatment.[353]

A study that included 78 adult patients also found that a fish oil supplement was significantly more effective than a placebo at preventing relapses of Crohn's. Over the course of the year, 28% of the patients who received the supplement relapsed, compared with 69% of those who received the placebo.[354]

Unfortunately, three larger randomized studies (including 135, 374, and 379 patients, respectively), found that adults with Crohn's who received fish oil capsules were just as likely to relapse as those who received a placebo.[355] An additional study found that three months of treatment with fish oil wasn't significantly different than a placebo in its effects on disease activity and its ability to heal the intestinal mucosa.[356]

Why such divergent results? One possibility might be the type of fish oil capsules that were used. In both of the placebo-controlled studies that found fish oil beneficial, the oil was contained in specially coated capsules that were designed to release their contents in the small intestine rather than the stomach.[357] Soft gelatin capsules that break down in the stomach were used in the studies showing no benefit from fish oil.

Might fish oil be more effective when it is released in the small intestine rather than broken down in the stomach?[358] We don't know for sure. It is absorbed by the body regardless of where it is released, so it's hard to explain why this might make a difference.

The verdict? The jury is still out on whether adding fish or fish oil to your diet might have some value in maintaining remission from Crohn's.

# Looking toward the plant world

We've looked to the oceans; maybe it's time to explore the green places of the earth for something that could make a difference for people with Crohn's. Curcumin, wormwood, and aloe all have their advocates.

## Curcumin

These days those who are curious about nutritional supplements are starting to hear more about curcumin, a compound found in the plant *Curcuma longa*. Curcumin is known primarily as the main pigment in turmeric, a spice widely used in South Asian cuisines. But preliminary research has also suggested that curcumin might have some immunosuppressive and anti-inflammatory effects.[359]

Could curcumin be useful in Crohn's disease? So far it has only been tested in two small studies. One included 27 patients with IBD who were dependent on steroids: 16 with ulcerative colitis, and 11 with Crohn's. A Curcuma extract wasn't any more effective than a placebo in helping the patients reduce their steroid dose.[360]

Another study of curcumin in IBD patients included five participants with Crohn's. The patients took a curcumin supplement for two months while continuing with their usual medications. One had a fistula that got a little worse. The remaining four had decreases in disease activity and ESR.[361] But because there wasn't a comparison group of patients who weren't taking curcumin, there is no way to know if the improvement was due to the standard medical treatment or the supplement. For the moment, it remains unclear whether curcumin offers any special benefits for people with Crohn's.

## Wormwood

The herb wormwood (*Artemisia absinthium pulvis*) is best known as a component of the liqueur absinthe, the potent drink so popular among avante-garde writers and artists in the nineteenth and early twentieth centuries. But wormwood has also been used in folk medicine since ancient times. Its essential oil may have some antifungal, antiparasitic, and antimicrobial activity.[362] Wormwood has been assessed recently for its potential value in treating Crohn's.

Forty Crohn's patients who were using steroids were randomly assigned to receive wormwood capsules or a placebo for 10 weeks. They tapered and discontinued their steroids over the course of the study. Only 2 of the 20 patients who received wormwood developed worsening Crohn's symptoms during the steroid taper, compared with 16 of the 20 who received the placebo. Fewer patients in the wormwood group had to restart steroids (only 2 patients versus 11 in the placebo group). The positive effects of wormwood seemed to continue for several weeks after the supplement was discontinued.[363]

It will be interesting to see if these effects can be duplicated in larger studies. But for the moment it would be unwise to embark on a wormwood regimen outside of a carefully supervised clinical trial.

❖ **Wormwood can cause seizures and other toxic effects on the nervous system.**[364]

We need to know much more about its potential risks and benefits before considering its use for people with Crohn's.

## Aloe

Occasionally people ask whether products made from a plant called
aloe vera can help control Crohn's disease. But there aren't any published studies of aloe in people with Crohn's and it would be wise
to be cautious about supplements that contain it. Aloe was once
used as an ingredient in laxatives. Taken orally, it can cause abdominal cramps and diarrhea—not welcome side effects if you have
Crohn's![365]

# Food-exclusion diets:
# are they worth the effort?

Another dietary option we haven't yet considered is developing a
personalized diet by testing foods individually and avoiding those
that cause symptoms. A couple of studies have suggested that this
type of food testing and exclusion might help people with Crohn's
disease stay in remission longer. Others seem to indicate little benefit. Let's take a closer look.

In one small study, patients who had just achieved remission
from Crohn's disease using TPN or total enteral nutrition adopted
a diet rich in fiber and unrefined carbohydrates or reintroduced
food gradually to identify items that caused symptoms. Among
10 patients assigned to the high-fiber diet, 8 relapsed within two
months and the remaining 2 within six months. In comparison, 7 of
10 patients who introduced foods one by one were still in remission
at six months on their personally developed food-exclusion diet.[366]

The poor results with the high-fiber diet are surprising since
we've just seen that the amount of dietary fiber doesn't seem to

make much difference in the course of Crohn's. The authors don't say how the high-fiber diet was introduced. If it was started all at once in these patients who had been using a liquid diet or TPN instead of building up the amount of fiber over a week or two, that could have accounted for some quick relapses.

The same food-exclusion protocol was tested in a larger series of 77 patients with Crohn's. The participants used TPN, total enteral nutrition, or an exclusion diet until they were in remission, and then reintroduced one food per day, supplementing their diet with an elemental formula until they had added enough foods to constitute a nutritionally adequate diet. Any food that produced symptoms was retested at the end of the food-reintroduction protocol and added to or eliminated from the diet depending on the results of the retest.

Patients then followed their personalized diet on a long-term basis, avoiding any foods that had caused symptoms during the testing process. If they developed symptoms, they were told to use only an elemental diet and spring water for three to four days, and then return carefully to their personal diet. At the end of the year, 52 of the 77 patients were still in remission, decreasing to 26 at the end of two years, and 18 at the end of three years.[367]

This study has two weaknesses. First, there wasn't a control group of patients following a normal diet, so we don't know if the patients would have done just as well without using an exclusion diet. Second, the patients testing the food-exclusion diet were told to switch to an elemental diet whenever they started to develop symptoms, so it's unclear whether the sustained remission they achieved was due to the food-exclusion protocol or to the short courses of enteral nutrition. The author doesn't indicate how many patients needed to switch over to the elemental diet temporarily or how often they had to do so.

Luckily another study is available that can help us better assess the value of food-exclusion diets. Thirty-three adults with Crohn's were randomly assigned to follow a food-testing protocol or a high-fiber diet for a year. Those in the high-fiber group were asked to eat fruits and vegetables, reduce their refined sugar consumption, and replace other refined carbohydrates such as white flour and white rice with whole grain flours and brown rice. Some spontaneously avoided certain foods on their own that they considered caused them symptoms—most commonly sauerkraut, milk, orange juice, and pulses (plants with edible seeds such as lentils, chickpeas, kidney beans, etc.).

The patients assigned to the food-testing regimen had a more complicated task. They introduced foods to their diet at the rate of one every two days, supplementing their meals with an elemental formula until they had added enough foods to constitute a nutritionally adequate diet. If a food did not produce symptoms when introduced, it was eaten as desired from then onwards. If symptoms did occur, the patient returned to safe foods until symptom-free, and waited to retest the problem food until the end of the food-reintroduction protocol. At that point, depending on the results of the retest, the food was accepted as a safe or designated as a product to avoid. Once all of the testing was completed, patients were told to continue to avoid their problem foods for the remainder of the year.

❖ **Disease activity was similar over the course of the year regardless of whether the patients followed the food-testing protocol or the high-fiber diet.**

It didn't matter whether the patients began the trial with chronically active Crohn's disease or disease in remission; they still did equally well with the two diets.[368] It's true that some of the patients using the high-fiber diet excluded some foods on their own, but going through the tedious food-testing process didn't offer any additional benefits.

Another study evaluating a food-exclusion regimen also found that the process was of relatively limited utility. This trial included 42 patients with Crohn's who had gone into remission using an elemental diet. An individualized food-reintroduction program was designed for each person, taking into account foods they felt had given them problems in the past and reserving those items to test last. One food was introduced every five days, with the elemental diet continued as a nutritional supplement until enough foods had been added to constitute an adequate diet. Foods identified as problematic after at least two attempts were investigated at the end in a double-blind fashion (with neither patient nor doctor knowing whether a series of test meals contained the food).

Out of the 42 patients, only 5 were definitively proven intolerant to specific foods in the double-blind challenges (and to only one food each). A sixth patient was identified as lactose-intolerant based on a lactose tolerance test, and a seventh identified a potential food sensitivity (alcohol) that could not be tested in a double-blind fashion.[369]

Another food-testing study that included a double-blind phase also found few verifiable food intolerances. Twenty-seven patients who achieved remission on enteral nutrition were offered the choice of reintroducing normal food gradually or testing one new food per day instead. For the 20 patients who went through the food-testing regimen, any food identifying as triggering problems was tested again at the end in a double-blind fashion.

Six patients relapsed early in the food-testing process and required steroid treatment or surgery. Of the 14 able to complete the regimen, 5 didn't identify any problematic foods. Four others identified items that they felt caused symptoms, but none of the foods caused problems in double-blind tests. The remaining 5 patients identified potential trigger foods, but refused to undergo double-blind testing.

Overall, disease location, rather than whether a patient went through food testing or not, was the only significant predictor of relapse. Among the patients with colonic disease, with or without small intestinal involvement, 80% relapsed within six months of completing their course of total enteral nutrition, compared with 27% of those whose disease was limited to the small intestine.[370]

Is it worth spending weeks slowly adding foods to your diet to achieve this relatively low likelihood of identifying a problematic item? Only you can decide.

## If you want to try food testing . . .

If you want to experiment with a food-testing regimen to try to find out whether particular foods trigger symptoms for you, there are a variety of possible approaches. You could introduce one food per day or every other day, or even every fourth or fifth day if you want to be particularly careful. Or you could follow one of various food-reintroduction protocols that others have used in the past.

One protocol you might consider was developed at Addenbrooke's Hospital in Cambridge (UK). The diet calls for introducing one new food a day, and eating it in generous helpings two or three times during the day. If the food doesn't cause any symptoms, it can be eaten freely from then on. But if a possible reaction is noted, the item is removed from the diet and rechallenged later for four days. Cereal grains (wheat, rye, barley, etc.) are tested for up to seven days. Two rest days with no new food introductions follow every seven days of food testing in case any of the foods cause delayed reactions. Patients keep a diary of everything they eat and any symptoms they observe to make it easier to identify the cause of any reactions that might occur. They continue to use enteral nutrition during the testing process until they are eating enough different foods to constitute a balanced diet.

If any food provokes a severe reaction, patients don't test any other foods until they are symptom-free again. If necessary, they may restart total enteral nutrition for two or three days until the symptoms pass. Once the testing process is complete, they stay on the resulting diet until two or three years have passed without symptoms before retrying foods that previously provoked reactions.[371]

In a study that used this protocol, foods were introduced in the following order: lamb, pears, rice, broccoli, white fish, carrots, turkey, tomatoes, beef, tap water, banana, milk, peas, tea, cabbage, apple, chicken, pork, yeast tablets, potatoes, butter, eggs, wheat, coffee beans, leeks, cane sugar, white wine, oranges, brussels sprouts, beet sugar, lettuce, corn, onion, parsnips, cheddar cheese, mushrooms, white bread, spinach, grapefruit, plain chocolate, grapes, courgettes or marrow, soy beans, cauliflower, oats, rhubarb, instant coffee, honey, melon, celery, lemon, olive oil, turnip or rutabaga, yogurt, white bread, monosodium glutamate, prawns or shrimps, and saccharine tablets.[372] A later publication offers a different sequence, with the first 30 foods introduced being chicken, rice, pears, soy margarine, soy milk, carrots, potatoes, white fish, runner beans, cooking oil, bananas, turkey, peas, milk, cheese, tea, beef, apple, lamb, cauliflower, tomatoes, mushrooms, eggs, butter/margarine, onions, oranges, yogurt, wheat, yeast, bread.[373]

## Another approach to food testing

Those who would prefer a speedier approach to food testing might appreciate an alternative protocol developed at the same hospital. Patients using the abbreviated protocol move directly from total enteral nutrition to a low-fiber, fat-limited ("LOFFLEX") diet that excludes food products that have frequently been reported to cause symptoms by patients with Crohn's. The LOFFLEX diet allows the following:

- all fish, shellfish, lean meat, and poultry except pork, fish cooked in batter or breading, and fish canned in oil or tomato sauce
- two portions a day of any vegetables prepared without skins, seeds, or stalks, with the exception of pulses (peas and beans), onions, tomatoes, and sweet corn
- two portions a day of any fruit prepared without skins or seeds, but not citrus fruits, dried fruits, apples, or bananas
- soy milk and soy products, with soy margarine in moderation
- rice, rice cakes, Rice Krispies, tapioca, sago, and arrowroot.
- sunflower and olive oils in moderation, but no corn or vegetable oils
- salt, pepper, herbs, spices, sugar, honey, and jam
- tap water, mineral water, fruit and herbal teas, non-citrus fruit juices, and Ribena.

After two weeks on this limited diet (or four weeks for those who develop any symptoms), additional foods are added one at a time and tested for four days each, with the exception of wheat products, which are tested for seven days. Each food that does not provoke symptoms is added to the initial restricted diet.

The advantage of this method is that you can move directly to a varied diet of solid food and have fewer food products to test individually. In a study comparing it with standard food testing (introducing one food at a time), the LOFFLEX protocol was equally effective at maintaining remission (although the patients chose which dietary protocol they would use rather than being randomly assigned).[374]

On the other hand, the LOFFLEX protocol has not been tested to see whether it decreases the risk of relapse in people with Crohn's compared with adopting a normal, unrestricted diet. So far no conclusive evidence proves that *any* food-testing regimen lengthens remission compared with an unselected diet. But indisputably some people find that watching their diet can make a real difference. If you're one of them, you may find these protocols useful guides as you strive to identify your own ideal diet.

# Is lactose a problem?

When people think about excluding items from their diet in the hope of getting better control of Crohn's, many decide to avoid dairy products containing lactose. As we learned in Chapter 7, lactose is the carbohydrate found in milk. When we drink milk, an enzyme in our body called **lactase** breaks down the lactose into simple sugars that are easily absorbed by the small intestine.[375] Some people aren't as good as others at absorbing lactose because they have lower levels of lactase.

Are people with Crohn's likely to have trouble digesting lactose? You'll often hear casual advice to avoid dairy products from fellow patients with IBD. But although some studies indicate that people with Crohn's disease are more likely to be lactose-intolerant than the general population, other studies haven't found any differences.[376]

*However*, when someone is having a flare-up of Crohn's, they may be more likely to have trouble digesting lactose than when the disease is in remission.[377] There are also at least some data suggesting that lactose intolerance may be more common in patients with small intestinal Crohn's disease than in those with Crohn's colitis.[378] That wouldn't be a big surprise, since lactose is broken down and absorbed in the small intestine and damage to the small intestine could interfere with that process.

If you suspect that you may have difficulty absorbing lactose, you can take a screening test called a hydrogen breath test to find out. But don't assume that you need to avoid dairy products just because you have Crohn's. Many people with Crohn's have normal lactose absorption, especially if they're in remission. Also, even people who are lactose-intolerant can often consume small amounts of dairy products without problems. Most double-blind studies have found that the majority of healthy people who test positive for lactose malabsorption can consume at least a cup of milk without symptoms—even people who are convinced they can't tolerate even the tiniest amounts of dairy products.[379]

That said, there are a handful of reports of people with Crohn's who do not have a clear milk protein allergy or lactose intolerance, but still do not seem to tolerate milk.[380] But these cases are the exception rather than the rule. As long as you don't have a severe reaction from consuming milk, don't feel you need to pass up dairy products.

Unnecessarily steering clear of dairy can have some real disadvantages. Individuals who consider themselves intolerant of milk have significantly lower bone density than those who do not report any problems with milk consumption.[381] If you do exclude milk and cheese from your diet, make sure to consume enough calcium from other dietary sources or supplements to maintain strong and healthy bones.

## What about probiotics?

**Probiotics** are microorganisms that may be beneficial to their hosts and are nonpathogenic, meaning that they do not normally cause disease. Naturally occurring probiotics have been around for centuries. They are present in a wide variety of fermented food products—everything from the familiar yogurt to a Central Asian milk drink called kefir.[382]

Probiotics are sometimes prescribed for patients who have to take strong antibiotics or have severe diarrhea. They are used to help restore "good" intestinal bacteria that might have been wiped out by antibiotics or diarrheal conditions.[383] In people with ulcerative colitis, probiotics seem to help prevent pouchitis (i.e., inflammation of the internal pouch created to collect waste after removal of the colon and rectum).[384]

Unfortunately probiotics don't appear to have any particular benefit in people with Crohn's. A very small study (including only four children!) suggested that a probiotic bacterium called *Lactobacillus* GG might potentially be beneficial.[385] But three larger, randomized trials showed that *Lactobacillus* GG wasn't any more effective than a placebo in helping children or adults with Crohn's maintain remission.[386]

Two other randomized studies tested a different *Lactobacillus* species with equally disappointing results. *Lactobacillus johnsonii* LA1 was no more effective than a placebo at preventing disease recurrence.[387]

Success was equally elusive in a randomized study of a probiotic product called Mutaflor that contains a nonpathogenic strain of *Escherichia coli* (strain Nissle 1917). Although the hope was that this probiotic might compete with pathogenic (disease-causing) forms of *E. coli* in the colon and suppress their growth, it was no more useful than a placebo in a one-year study.[388]

Several other studies of probiotics have been performed in patients with Crohn's (testing VSL#3 or *Saccharomyces boulardii*), but they offer little useful data since the studies were poorly designed or had many dropouts.[389] Given the available evidence, it is not surprising that a systematic review of studies of probiotics found no evidence that they were effective at maintaining remission in people with Crohn's.[390]

Remember that some 400 to 500 different bacterial strains are happily inhabiting your intestines at any given moment.[391] A probiotic containing a single bacterial strain or even half a dozen is up against a lot of competition!

## A warning about probiotics

Probiotic use is not entirely risk-free. The bacteria used in probiotics don't cause disease if they stay where they belong in the intestinal tract. And this is virtually always where they stay. But if a probiotic moves through the walls of the intestines and gets into the blood, it is possible for it to cause a dangerous fungal infection.

Normally this never occurs. But a handful of cases of fungal infections thought to be caused by probiotics have been reported, chiefly in elderly people, people using catheters, or those with short bowel syndrome or compromised immune systems (whether because of an autoimmune condition like IBD or the use of immunomodulating drugs).[392] The risk is probably exceedingly small, and concentrated in seriously ill individuals, but it is worth knowing that it does exist.

# Prebiotics: a newer approach

**Prebiotics** contain one or more types of fiber found naturally in over 36,000 species of plants, including many that we eat on a regular basis—onions, garlic, bananas, and wheat, for instance. Because prebiotics aren't absorbed by the body, they are used to add fiber to foods without adding calories.[393] In theory, when prebiotics are fermented in the gastrointestinal tract, they might stimulate the growth of "good" bacteria in the intestines.

So far, only two studies have tested prebiotics in patients with Crohn's disease. In one small study, there were some mild improvements in disease activity when 10 patients with colonic or ileocolonic Crohn's disease added a prebiotic (Prebio 1) to their diet for three weeks. However, without an untreated comparison group it's hard to tell whether the improvement was due to the prebiotic or was simply a temporary placebo effect.[394]

An even smaller study (including two patients with Crohn's and five with ulcerative colitis) showed that 14 days' consumption of a prebiotic could lead to the appearance of *Bifidobacteria* (a "good" bacteria) in the feces of patients in whom the bacterium was not present before treatment. But the study was far too small to draw any conclusions about whether this change made any difference in the course of IBD. One of the patients with Crohn's had fewer and firmer bowel movements during the prebiotic treatment. The other developed blood in the stool.[395]

All in all, it's too early to tell whether prebiotics will have any special benefit in Crohn's. But you can get prebiotics without taking any special supplements. All you have to do is eat veggies and whole grains!

## What about synbiotics?

A **synbiotic** is a combination product containing both probiotics and prebiotics. So far, only one study has tested a synbiotic in people with Crohn's disease. Used for two years, Synbiotic 2000 wasn't any more effective than a placebo in maintaining remission in 30 patients who had just undergone resection surgery.[396]

## The Specific Carbohydrate Diet: does it really work?

The Specific Carbohydrate Diet is almost always mentioned when people ask about nutritional treatments for IBD. Some people rave about it, others dismiss it, but it certainly has more popular recognition than most other dietary options for gastrointestinal disease. The rules of this diet call for avoiding *all* cereal grains (no bread, pasta, oatmeal, rice, etc.), as well as many legumes, tubers such as potatoes and yams, sweeteners (except honey, saccharin, and sugars found in fruit and fruit juices), many dairy products (including milk and commercially manufactured yogurt), and a number of other miscellaneous items.[397]

In spite of the publicity that the Specific Carbohydrate Diet has received, a search of the medical literature reveals not a single published study testing this diet in people with Crohn's disease. Until and unless such studies are conducted, we have no way of knowing if the Specific Carbohydrate Diet offers any special benefit to people with Crohn's. But we've already seen that it doesn't make much difference whether you follow a high- or low-fiber diet, or restrict carbohydrates or sugar and yeast. It seems unlikely that the dietary manipulations dictated by the Specific Carbohydrate Diet would be any more likely to make a difference. Nevertheless, in the absence of medical evidence, it remains for you, the reader, to decide.

## The benefits of a well-balanced diet (Mom was right!)

It is undeniable that certain patients report remarkable success with nutritional regimens that haven't been clinically tested, such as the Specific Carbohydrate Diet, the Maker's Diet, or others. It's possible that their success lies not so much in the details of the specific diet they choose, but rather that by following a detailed dietary plan they end up consuming more nutritious foods than before. A regimen rich in fruits, vegetables, and whole grains offers far more of the vitamins and minerals that people with Crohn's may lack than a diet centered around white bread, pasta, pastries, and fast food. In addition, vegetables, fruits, and whole grains supply fiber, which can help bulk up stool in people prone to diarrhea and increase regularity in those with constipation.

At least one study has found that helping patients with Crohn's eat more nutritious foods has clear benefits. The study included 137 patients with Crohn's disease who were randomly assigned to two groups. One group didn't receive any counseling about nutrition.

The other received six months of dietary counseling (one session per month). There was no attempt to prescribe a one-size-fits-all regimen. Dietitians assessed each patient, and made individualized suggestions based on a given person's weight, nutrient intake, and dietary deficiencies.

At the end of the six months, those who received dietary advice, compared with those who didn't, had significantly better scores on a Crohn's disease activity index, had spent fewer days in the hospital due to Crohn's, and had missed significantly fewer days from work due to the disease. They were also more likely to be consuming the recommended dietary allowances of protein, riboflavin, and vitamin C.[398]

All in all, for those with Crohn's, what seems to matter most is avoiding nutritional deficiencies rather than the particular diet used to prevent them. If you have trouble eating a balanced diet, a meeting or two with a registered dietitian may help you develop a more satisfactory eating plan.

## WHAT HAVE WE LEARNED?

❖ Eating right for patients with Crohn's involves fewer dietary restrictions than many people fear. In general, those who prefer high-fiber or low-fiber diets don't have to worry that their preference will worsen their disease. Most Crohn's patients who enjoy dairy products can continue to consume them without anxiety.

❖ Low-carb and low-yeast diets aren't necessary.

❖ Supplements such as probiotics, prebiotics, synbiotics, and fish oil don't seem to have much effect on the course of the disease. However, eating a balanced diet and avoiding nutritional deficits may be helpful.

It is disappointing to see how little we can do to control Crohn's disease from a dietary standpoint, aside from the use of enteral nutrition. But it is still worth knowing what doesn't work. A survey of Canadian patients with IBD performed several years ago found that nearly half of those who used complementary and alternative medicine spent more than $250 a year on it.[399] Given the cost of treating a chronic disease like Crohn's, we need to know what really makes a difference so we avoid wasting our money on things that don't.

# APPENDIX A

❖

# Understanding
# Growth Charts

## How Does My Child Measure Up?

How does your child's height and weight compare with that of his or her peers? The growth charts on the following pages will help you find out.

The first two charts (one for girls and one for boys) show stature-for-age percentiles. The curved lines on the charts show the percentage of children in the US who are a given height at a given age.

For example, take a look at the chart for girls. Imagine that you have a 10-year-old daughter who is 4'6" tall. Find her height in inches (54") along the left edge of the table, and her age (10) along the bottom of the table, and look for the point where the two lines meet. That point falls just below the 50th percentile line (the curving percentile lines are labeled at their ends close to the right edge of the table). Your daughter is in approximately the 50th percentile for height, meaning that she is taller than half her peers, and shorter than the other half.

In contrast, a child 4'6" tall who was only nine years old would be in the 75th percentile of height among all US girls, i.e., taller than 75% of her peers. A 4'6" 12-year-old would be in the 3rd percentile of height, shorter than 97% of her peers.

The second two charts (one for girls and one for boys) show weight-for-age percentiles. The curved lines indicate the percentage of US children who are a given weight at a given age.

Find your child's weight along the left side of the table and his or her age along the bottom of the table and locate the point where the two lines meet. For instance, your 4'6" 10-year-old might weigh 58 pounds. The point where her age and weight meet on the chart for girls falls along the 10th percentile line. So she is only in the 10th percentile for weight, even though she is in the 50th percentile of height. She may be underweight.

But being in a low percentile for height or weight is not necessarily a problem. A child whose parents are both short might stay at the 15th percentile for height and weight throughout her growing years. The time to worry is when a child who has been stable at a given percentile falls into a lower percentile and stays there: falling from the 25th percentile to the 5th percentile, for example. That can be a signal that he or she is no longer growing at a normal pace. Consistently being in an unusually low percentile can also be a sign of trouble. A value below the 3rd percentile for height is sometimes considered an indicator of growth failure.

## CDC Growth Charts: United States

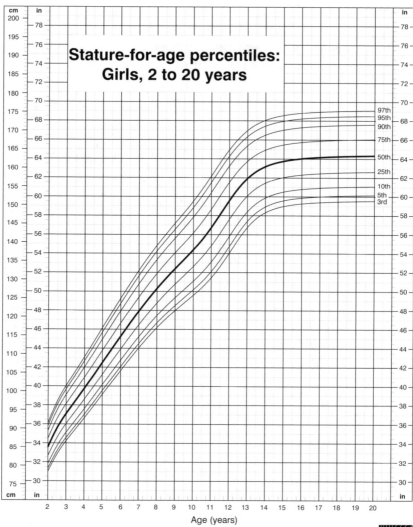

**Stature-for-age percentiles:
Girls, 2 to 20 years**

Age (years)

Published May 30, 2000.
SOURCE: Developed by the National Center for Health Statistics in collaboration with
the National Center for Chronic Disease Prevention and Health Promotion (2000).

SAFER·HEALTHIER·PEOPLE™

# CDC Growth Charts: United States

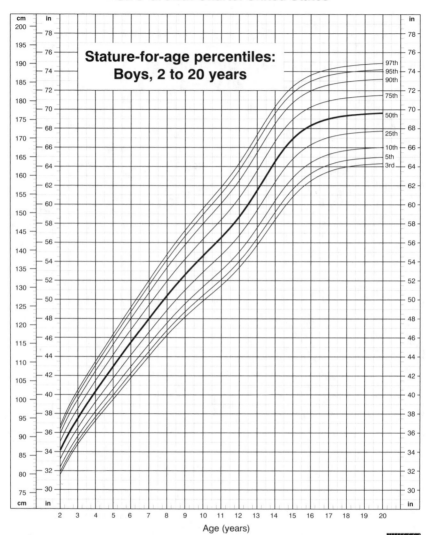

Stature-for-age percentiles:
Boys, 2 to 20 years

Age (years)

Published May 30, 2000.
SOURCE: Developed by the National Center for Health Statistics in collaboration with
the National Center for Chronic Disease Prevention and Health Promotion (2000).

SAFER·HEALTHIER·PEOPLE™

## CDC Growth Charts: United States

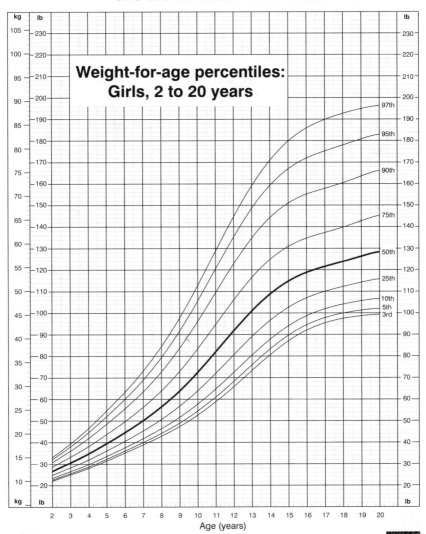

**Weight-for-age percentiles:
Girls, 2 to 20 years**

Age (years)

Published May 30, 2000.
SOURCE: Developed by the National Center for Health Statistics in collaboration with
the National Center for Chronic Disease Prevention and Health Promotion (2000).

SAFER·HEALTHIER·PEOPLE™

# CDC Growth Charts: United States

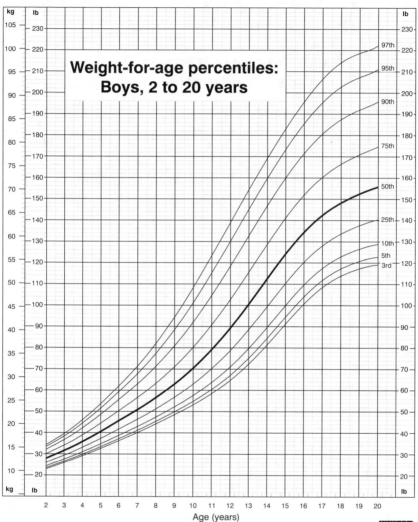

**Weight-for-age percentiles: Boys, 2 to 20 years**

Published May 30, 2000.
SOURCE: Developed by the National Center for Health Statistics in collaboration with
the National Center for Chronic Disease Prevention and Health Promotion (2000).

SAFER · HEALTHIER · PEOPLE™

# APPENDIX B

# Sources for Enteral Nutrition Formulas

The following companies make enteral nutrition products for adults and children. The list is not exhaustive—enteral nutrition formulas are available from many other manufacturers—but these are some of the major players.

Abbott Nutrition
Abbott Nutrition Consumer Relations
625 Cleveland Avenue
Columbus, Ohio 43215-1724
Tel. 1-800-227-5767
http://abbottnutrition.com

Abbott Nutrition
8401 Trans-Canada Highway
Saint-Laurent, Québec, Canada  H4S 1Z1
Tel. 1-800-361-7852
http://www.abbottnutrition.ca

Ajinomoto Co., Inc.
15-1, Kyobashi, 1-chome, Chuo-ku
Tokyo 104-8315 Japan
Tel. +81(3)5250-8111
www.ajinomoto.com

Fresenius Kabi AG
Corporate Communications
61346 Bad Homburg v.d.H.
Germany
Tel. +49 (0) 6172 686 0
www.fresenius-kabi.com

Lactalis Nutrition Santé
Parc d'activités de Torcé - Secteur Est – F
35370 TORCE
France
www.dhn.fr

Nestlé HealthCare Nutrition
25 Sheppard Ave West
North York
Ontario M2N 6S8
Canada
Tel. 1-800-565-1871
www.nutrition.nestle.ca

Nestlé Nutrition
800 N. Brand Boulevard, 9th Floor
Glendale, CA 91203
Tel. 1-800-422-2752
www.nestle-nutrition.com

Nutricia Clinical Care
White Horse Business Park
Trowbridge
Wiltshire
BA14 0XQ
Tel. 01225 751098
www.nutricia-clinical-care.uk

Nutricia North America
P.O. Box 117
Gaithersburg, MD 20884
Tel. 1-800-365-7354
www.shsna.com

Pfrimmer Nutricia GmbH
Am Weichselgarten 23
D-91058 Erlangen
Germany
Tel. 0800 688 742 42
www.pfrimmer-nutricia.de

SHS International Ltd.
100 Wavertree Blvd.
Liverpool L7 9PT
UK
Tel. +44 (0)151 228 8161
www.shs-nutrition.com

# NOTES

## Chapter 1

1. Levine, Milo, et al., 2003; Payne-James and Silk, 1990.
2. Hiwatashi, 1997; Ogata and Hibi, 2003.
3. Payne-James and Silk, 1990.
4. Blackburn et al., 1985.
5. Blackburn et al., 1985.
6. Greenstein et al., 1957.
7. Couch et al., 1960; Stephens et al., 1969.
8. Winitz, Seedman, and Graff, 1970.
9. Winitz et al., 1965.
10. Winitz et al., 1965.
11. Stephens et al, 1968; Thompson et al., 1969; Raith and Raith, 1989.
12. Stephens et al., 1968; Stephens et al., 1969; Thompson et al., 1969.
13. Stephens et al., 1969; Bounous et al., 1974.
14. E.g., Voitk et al., 1973; Bounous et al., 1974; Ou Tim et al., 1976; Goode et al., 1976; Axelsson and Jarnum, "Assessment," 1977; Navarro et al., 1978; O'Moráin et al., 1980; Morin et al., 1980; Morin et al., 1982; O'Moráin, 1982; O'Moráin et al., 1983.
15. Hull, 1985.
16. Lochs, Egger-Schödl, Pötzi, et al., 1984; Alun Jones, 1987; Greenberg et al., 1988; Wright and Adler, 1990; Furukawa et al., 1997 (however,

this study of 132 patients was retrospective); Kobayashi et al., 1998. A total of 308 patients participated in these six studies, but 15 in the study by Greenberg and colleagues were randomized to intravenous nutrition plus a normal diet. Hence only 293 patients received either total parenteral or total enteral nutrition.

17. Stokes et al., 1988; Galandiuk et al., 1990.
18. Dolz et al., 1989; Godeberge et al., 1989; Abad-Lacruz et al., 1990.
19. Randall, 1990; O'Sullivan and O'Morain, 2004.
20. Winitz, Adams, et al., 1970.
21. Axelsson and Justesen, 1977; O'Moráin, 1990; Giaffer, Holdsworth, and Duerden, 1991.
22. Lionetti et al., 2005.
23. Silk, 2000 (comment by J.O. Hunter in the "Discussion").
24. O'Moráin et al., 1984; Silk, 2000.
25. Silk, 2000.
26. Ruuska et al., 1994.
27. Law et al., 1973; Green, 1999.
28. Polk et al., 1992.
29. Gorard et al., 1993 (improvement was similar in malnourished and nourished patients); Teahon, Pearson, Smith, and Bjarnason, 1995 (9 of the 19 patients in this study had normal nutritional status on beginning treatment).
30. Bannerjee et al., 2004.
31. Teahon, Pearson, Smith, and Bjarnason, 1995.
32. Jones et al., 1993; Breese et al., 1995; Arnott et al., 1997; Fell et al., 2000; Meister et al., 2002; Yamamoto et al., 2005; Yamamoto et al., 2006; de Jong et al., 2007.
33. Bodemar et al., 1991. Even supplemental enteral nutrition, using an average of only 550 calories per day of the supplement, has been reported to produce a small but significant reduction in orosomucoid levels by Harries et al., 1984.
34. Navarro et al., 1982; Le Quintrec et al., 1987; Okada et al., 1990; Grimaud et al., 1990; Rigaud et al., 1991; Beattie et al., 1994; Breese et al., 1994; Matsui et al., 1995; Fell et al., 2000; Afzal et al., 2004; Afzal et al., 2005; Yamamoto et al., 2005; Borrelli et al., 2006; Berni Canani et al., 2006; Yamamoto et al., 2006.
35. Mansfield et al., 1995; Davison et al., 1996.
36. Sanderson, Boulton, et al., 1987; Ito et al., 1992; Teahon, Smethurst, et al., 1991; Zoli et al., 1997; Iwata et al, 2001.

37. Stephens et al., 1972; Logan, Gillon, Ferrington, and Ferguson, 1981; Ferguson, Glen, and Ghosh, 1998.
38. Hannon et al., 2007.
39. Götze and Ptok, 1993.
40. Nelson et al., 1977; Russell and Hall, 1979.
41. Stehr et al., 1983; Polk et al., 1992; Thomas, Holly, et al., 1993; Beattie et al., 1998; Bannerjee et al., 2004.
42. Heuschkel, 2004.

## Chapter 2
43. Summers et al., 1979.
44. Van Hees et al., 1981.
45. Ewe et al., 1989; Lennard Jones, 1977; Malchow et al., 1984; Summers et al., 1979.
46. Summers et al., 1979; "Salazopyrin in the management of Crohn's disease," 1985.
47. Singleton et al., 1993; Thomsen et al., 1998.
48. Singleton et al., 1993; Singleton, 1994.
49. Not superior to placebo: Brignola et al., 1992; Thomson et al., 1995; de Franchis et al., 1997; Sutherland et al., 1997; Lochs et al., 2000; superior to placebo: Prantera et al., 1992; Arber et al., 1995; Brignola et al., 1995; McLeod et al., 1995.
50. Mahmud et al., 2001.
51. Gorard et al., 1993; González-Huiz, de Léon, et al., 1993; Seidman, Griffiths, et al., 1993.
52. Summers et al., 1979; Wright and Scott, 1997.
53. Lichtenstein, 2001.
54. Faubion et al., 2001.
55. Lichtenstein, 2001.
56. Semeao et al., 1999.
57. Greenberg et al., 1994; Rutgeerts et al., 1994; Gross at et al., 1996; Campieri et al., 1997; Thomsen et al., 1998; Bar-Meir et al., 1998; Tremaine et al., 2002; Escher et al., 2004; Tursi et al., 2006.
58. Rutgeerts et al., 1994; Gross et al., 1996; Campieri et al., 1997; Bar-Meir et al., 1998; Levine, Weizman, et al., 2003; Escher et al., 2004.
59. Greenberg et al., 1996; Löfberg et al, 1996; Gross at et al., 1998; Ferguson, Campieri, et al., 1998; Hellers et al., 1999; Ewe et al., 1999; Hanauer et al., 2005; Sandborn, Löfberg, et al., 2005.
60. Ursing et al., 1982.

61. Schneider et al., 1981; Schneider et al., 1985.
62. Palder et al., 1991; McKee and Keenan, 1996.
63. Brandt et al., 1982.
64. Brandt et al., 1982; Gugler et al., 1989.
65. Prantera et al., 1998; Colombel et al., 1999; Arnold et al., 2002.
66. Prantera et al., 1998.
67. Present et al., 1980; Perrault et al., 1991; Korelitz et al., 1993.
68. Korelitz et al., 1993.
69. Present et al., 1980.
70. Markowitz at et al., 2000.
71. Hanauer et al., 2004.
72. Present et al., 1980; Korelitz and Present, 1985; Markowitz at et al., 1990; Hinojosa et al., 1995.
73. Lewis at et al., 2001; Warman et al., 2003.
74. Wright et al., 2004.
75. Summers et al., 1979.
76. Candy et al., 1995.
77. Vilien et al., 2004.
78. O'Donoghue et al., 1978.
79. Chebli et al., 2007.
80. D'Haens et al., 1999.
81. Rankin et al., 1979; McKee and Keenan, 1996.
82. McKee and Keenan, 1996.
83. Lecomte et al., 2003. The title and abstract of this study indicate that the participants were taking either azathiaprine or 6-MP, but it is important to note that 92 of the 94 patients used azathioprine. Therefore the results cannot be generalized to draw any conclusions about 6-MP.
84. Oren et al., 1997; Arora et al., 1999.
85. Feagan et al., 1995.
86. Chong et al., 2001.
87. Lémann et al., 1996.
88. Feagan et al., 2000.
89. Mahadevan et al., 2003.
90. Ardizzone et al., 2003.
91. Maté-Jiménez et al., 2000.
92. Kugathasan et al., 2000; Borrelli et al., 2004; Orlando at et al., 2005; Hyams, Crandall, et al., 2007.
93. Ardizzone et al., 2002; Cezard et al., 2004; Lémann et al., 2006.

94. Hanauer et al., 2002; Lémann et al., 2006; Hyams, Crandall, et al., 2007.
95. Borrelli et al., 2004; Rutgeerts et al., 2006.
96. Rutgeerts et al., 2006.
97. Present et al., 1999; Ouraghi et al., 2001; Ardizzone et al., 2002; Ardizzone et al., 2004; Luna-Chadid et al., 2004; Sands et al., 2004.
98. Rasul et al., 2004; Lichtenstein et al., 2005.
99. Domènech et al., 2005.
100. Ouraghi et al., 2001.
101. Sandborn, Rutgeerts, et al., 2007.
102. Hanauer et al., 2006.
103. Sandborn, Hanauer, et al., 2007.
104. Colombel et al., 2007.
105. Hinojosa et al., 2007.
106. Hanauer, et al., 2006; Sandborn, Rutgeerts, et al., 2007.
107. Colombel et al., 2007.
108. Biogen Idec Inc., Form 8-K filed with the United States Securities and Exchange Commission July 31, 2008; available at http://www.sec.gov/Archives/edgar/data/875045/0000950 13508005223/b714958ke8vk.htm (accessed August 18, 2008).
109. Sandborn, Colombel, et al., 2005; Hyams, Wilson, et al., 2007; Targan et al., 2007.
110. Sandborn, Colombel, et al., 2005.
111. Sandborn, Feagan, et al., 2007.
112. Schreiber et al., 2007.
113. Sachar, 1990.
114. Sachar, 1990.
115. Alun Jones, 1987; Lochs et al., 1991; Seidman, Griffiths, et al., 1993; González-Huiz, de León, et al., 1993; Gassull et al., 2002.
116. Malchow et al., 1990; Lochs et al., 1991; Riordan et al., 1993; Middleton et al., 1995; Griffiths, Pendley, et al., 2000; Afzal et al., 2005.
117. Blair et al., 1986; Ginsberg and Albert, 1988; Ginsberg and Albert, "Treatment of Crohn's disease," 1989; Cosgrove and Jenkins, 1997.
118. Le Quintrec et al., 1987; O'Brien et al., 1991. The 63% figure comes from the study by O'Brien. The percentage reaching steroid-free remission in the study by Le Quintrec and colleagues is unclear. There were 18 patients, 2 of whom were treated twice. It appears that 11 unique patients (61%) achieved steroid-free remission at least in the

short term, and that in 9 courses of treatment, most likely representing 8 unique patients, those treated remained steroid-free for between 6 and 30 months.

119. Takazoe et al., 1995.
120. Navarro et al., 1978; Russell and Hall, 1979; Morin et al., 1982; Lochs, Egger-Schödl, Schuh et al., 1984; Teahon et al., 1990.
121. Le Quintrec et al., 1987; Rigaud et al., 1991; Beattie et al., 1994; Fell et al., 2000; Yamamoto et al., 2005.
122. Okada et al., 1990; Breese et al., 1994; Borrelli et al., 2006; Berni Canani et al., 2006.
123. Wilschanski et al., 1996; Verma, Kirkwood, et al., 2000.
124. Verma et al., 2001.
125. Kirschner et al., 1981; Werlin, 1981; Aiges et al., 1989; Israel and Hassall, 1995.

**Chapter 3**
126. Lochs et al., 2006.
127. Navarro et al., 1978; O'Moráin, 1979; Morin et al., 1980; Morin et al., 1982; O'Moráin, 1982; Stober et al., 1983; O'Moráin et al., 1983; Neidich et al., 1985.
128. O'Moráin et al., 1983.
129. Sarles, 1988.
130. Sanderson, Udeen, et al., 1987; Seidman, Lohoues, et al., 1991; Seidman, Griffiths, et al., 1993; Thomas, Taylor, and Miller, 1993; Ruuska et al., 1994; Borrelli et al., 2006.
131. Chafai et al., 1995; Papadopoulou et al., 1995.
132. Comité de nutrition de la Société française de pédiatrie, 2005 ("L'alimentation entérale exclusive représente une alternative efficace à la corticothérapie dans le traitement des poussées aiguës de la maladie de Crohn, en particulier en cas de dénutrition").
133. Sanderson, Udeen, et al., 1987; Seidman, Lohoues, et al., 1991; Seidman, Griffiths, et al., 1993.
134. Sanderson, Udeen, et al., 1987; Seidman, Lohoues, et al., 1991; Thomas, Taylor, and Miller, 1993.
135. Griffiths et al., 2000; Afzal et al., 2005.
136. The 65-child study (Afzal et al., 2005) excluded children with strictures, recent use of steroids or immunomodulating drugs, or current use of antibiotics. Because strictures can be difficult to treat with enteral nutrition, and antibiotics are often used in the presence of

perianal disease, which is also difficult to treat with liquid diets, these exclusion criteria probably resulted a study population that was more responsive to enteral nutrition than an unselected group of children with Crohn's. The 84-child study (Griffiths et al., 2000) was published only as an abstract, and no exclusion/inclusion criteria are provided, except that the participants could have either new or relapsing small and/or large intestinal Crohn's. The study compared two different enteral nutrition formulas, which were not significantly different in their ability to induce remission (62% remission rate with one formula, 52% with the other). The 57% remission rate that I cite reflects the total number of patients achieving remission (48/84), regardless of the formula used.

137. Unless otherwise specified, here and in the other personal stories in this book, names have been changed to protect the privacy of contributors.
138. Sanderson, Udeen, et al., 1987; Thomas, Taylor, and Miller, 1993; Chafai et al., 1995; Papadopoulou et al., 1995; Seidman et al., 1996; Berni Canani et al., 2006.
139. Chafai et al., 1995.
140. Sanderson, Udeen, et al., 1987.
141. Saint-Raymond et al., 1988.
142. Walker-Smith, 1996.
143. Seidman, LeLeiko, et al., 1991; Sentongo et al., 2000.
144. Seidman, LeLeiko, et al., 1991; Markowitz et al., 1993; Sentongo et al., 2000.
145. Markowitz et al., 1993.
146. Michener and Wyllie, 1990.
147. Akobeng et al., 2002.
148. Borrelli et al., 2006.
149. Breese et al., 1994.
150. Berni Canani et al., 2006.
151. Beattie et al., 1994; Fell et al., 2000.
152. Modigliani et al., 1990; Olaison et al., 1990; Breese et al., 1994; Borrelli et al., 2006.
153. Cosgrove and Jenkins, 1997.
154. Blair et al., 1986.
155. Saint-Raymond et al., 1988.
156. Randell and Murphy, 2001.
157. Knight et al., 2005.
158. Saint-Raymond et al., 1988.

159. Fujimura et al., 1992.
160. Belli et al., 1988; Polk et al., 1992; Seidman et al., 1996.
161. Belli et al., 1988.
162. Polk et al., 1992.
163. Belli et al., 1988; Polk et al., 1992.
164. Wilschanski et al., 1996. Also see Navarro et al., 1982, for a report on 17 children with Crohn's who used total enteral nutrition for 2 to 7 months, and then used the formula to supply 50% of their calories for an additional 12 to 22 months.
165. Aiges et al., 1989; Israel and Hassall, 1995; Cosgrove and Jenkins, 1997.
166. Werlin, 1981.
167. Werlin, 1981.
168. Kirschner et al., 1981.
169. Johnson et al., 2006.
170. Aiges et al., 1989.
171. Motil, Grand, Maletskos, and Young, 1982.
172. Seidman, Griffiths, et al., 1993; Day et al., 2006.
173. Griffiths, 2005.
174. Afzal et al., 2005.
175. Wilschanski et al., 1996.
176. Papadopoulou et al., 1995; Day et al., 2006.
177. Papadopoulou et al., 1995.
178. Knight et al., 2005.
179. Thomas, Taylor, and Miller, 1993.
180. E.g., Cucchiara et al., 1984.
181. Rabbett et al., 1996.
182. Wilschanski et al., 1996.
183. Gailhoustet et al., 2002.
184. Afzal et al., 2004.

**Chapter 4**
185. Giaffer, Holdsworth, and Duerden, 1991.
186. Riordan et al., 1993.
187. Jones et al., 1993.
188. O'Brien et al., 1991.
189. Yamamoto et al., 2005.
190. Grimaud et al., 1990.
191. Fukuda et al., 1995.

192. O'Moráin et al., 1984; González-Huix, de León, et al., 1993; Zoli et al., 1997.

193. Okada et al., 1990. This was a quasi-randomized trial. The first 10 patients were assigned to the enteral nutrition group and the second 10 to prednisolone.

194. Gorard et al., 1993.

195. Malchow et al., 1990.

196. Lochs et al., 1991.

197. Su et al., 2004.

198. Carter et al., 2004.

199. O'Brien et al., 1991.

200. Le Quintrec et al., 1987.

201. Ginsberg and Albert, 1988.

202. Ginsberg and Albert, "Treatment of Crohn's disease," 1989.

203. Okada et al., 1990.

204. Yamamoto et al., 2005.

205. Rigaud et al., 1991.

206. Grimaud et al., 1990.

207. Brignola et al., 1983; Harries et al., 1983; Harries et al., 1984.

208. Stein and the German Society for Digestive and Metabolic Diseases, 2003 ("Bei Vorliegen einer Malnutrition [gleichgültig, ob es sich um eine generelle Mangelernährung oder spezifische Mängel handelt] ist eine Supplementierung mit einer nährstoffdefinierten Kost [ca. 500 ml pro Tag] zu empfehlen").

209. Verma, Kirkwood, et al., 2000.

210. Verma et al., 2001.

211. Afdhal et al., 1989.

212. Takagi et al., 2006; Yamamoto, Nakahigashi, Saniabadi, et al., 2007; Yamamoto, Nakahigashi, Umegae, et al., 2007.

213. Ikeuchi et al., 2000; Ikeuchi et al., 2004.

214. Esaki et al, 2005; Esaki et al., 2006.

215. Hirakawa et al., 1993.

216. Lochs et al., 1984; Afdhal et al., 1989; Mansfield et al., 1995; Matsui et al., 1995.

217. Teahon et al., 1990; Gorard et al., 1993.

218. Mansfield et al., 1995; Matsui et al., 1995; Verma, Brown, et al., 2000.

219. Matsui et al., 1995.

220. Teahon et al., 1990. Also, Gorard et al., 1993, didn't find a difference in response between people with new-onset and established disease, and

González-Huix, de Léon, et al., 1993, and Verma, Brown, et al., 2000, found no association between disease location and response.

221. Rigaud et al., 1991.
222. Matsubayashi and Sanada, 1995.
223. Teahon, Pearson, et al., 1991.
224. Gorard et al., 1993.
225. Teahon, Pearson, Levi, and Bjarnason, 1995.

**Chapter 5**
226. Lim et al., 1998.
227. Cameron and Middleton, 2003.
228. Voitk et al., 1973; Göschke et al., 1977; Axelsson and Jarnum, "Elemental diet in gastrointestinal diseases," 1977; Calam et al., 1980; Morin et al., 1982; Rabast and Heskamp, 1986; Bret and Souquet, 1988.
229. Takazoe et al., 1995.
230. Calam et al., 1980.
231. Main et al., 1980.
232. Stephens et al., 1972; Giorgini et al., 1973. Also see Calam et al., 1980, reporting on the closure of two perianal fistulas in a patient who used total enteral nutrition for 14 weeks. The fistulas were still closed 20 months later. During the follow-up period the patient was also taking prednisolone and metronidazole maintenance therapy.
233. Berg and Classen, 1973.
234. E.g., Ou Tim et al., 1976.
235. Navarro et al., 1978.
236. Lochs, Egger-Schödl, Schuh, et al., 1984.
237. Morin et al., 1982.
238. Russell and Hall, 1979.
239. Fukuda et al., 1995.
240. Teahon et al., 1990.
241. Saint-Raymond et al., 1988; Younoszai, 1977.
242. Navarro et al., 1982; Sato et al., 1999; Yamamoto et al., 2006.
243. Navarro et al., 1982; Saint-Raymond et al., 1988.
244. Navarro et al., 1982.
245. Afdhal et al., 1989; Raouf et al., 1991; Woolner et al., 1998.
246. Baba and Nakai, 1995.
247. Thomas et al., 2000.
248. Thomas et al., 2000.
249. Heymsfield et al., 1983.

250. Heymsfield et al., 1983.
251. Poulin and Langevin, 1982.
252. Russell and Hall, 1979.
253. Jones et al., 2004.
254. McIntyre et al., 1983.
255. McIntyre et al., 1983.
256. Heymsfield et al., 1983.
257. Allison, 1986.
258. Main et al., 1980.
259. Navarro et al., 1982.
260. Sarles, 1988.
261. Triantafillidis et al., 2008.
262. Horie et al., 1997.
263. Harms et al., 2004.

**Chapter 6**
264. Stephens et al., 1969; Voitk et al., 1973; Ou Tim et al., 1976; Gassull et al., 1986.
265. E.g., Leenders et al., 1974.
266. Rocchio et al., 1974; Dickman et al., 1975; Klaassen et al., 1998; Meister et al., 2002.
267. Driscoll and Rosenberg, 1978.
268. Cezard and Messing, 1993.
269. Abad-Lacruz et al., 1990; González-Huix, Fernández-Bañares, et al, 1993; also see Rao et al., 1987, and Klaassen et al., 1998, for good toleration of enteral nutrition in colitis patients.
270. Abad-Lacruz et al., 1990; González-Huix, Fernández-Bañares, et al., 1993; Klaassen et al., 1998.
271. Greenberg et al., 1999.
272. Melmed et al., 2007.
273. Pimentel et al., 2000.
274. Burgmann et al., 2006.

**Chapter 7**
275. Fernández-Bañares et al., 1995; Griffiths et al., 1995; Zachos et al., 2007.
276. Giaffer et al., 1990 (two patients who didn't respond to a polymeric diet responded to an elemental diet); Raouf et al., 1991 (six responders switched from an elemental to a polymeric formula maintained their

improvement or improved further, four switched from a polymeric to an elemental formula maintained their improvement, and three switched from a polymeric to an elemental formula deteriorated significantly); Pearson et al., 1993 (three patients who were intolerant of an elemental formula responded to a modular formula); Royall et al., 1994 (a patient who did not respond to a semi-elemental diet responded to another elemental or semi-elemental formula); Mansfield et al., 1995 (a patient who improved slightly during 10 days of treatment with a semi-elemental diet made further improvement and reached remission after switching to an elemental diet); Woolner et al., 1998 (a patient didn't respond to one formula, but did respond to another; neither formula was identified).

277. Familydoctor.org editorial staff, "Food allergies: just the facts," American Academy of Family Physicians, Sep 2000, updated Nov 2005; available at http://familydoctor.org/online/famdocen/home /common/allergies/basics/340.html.html (accessed February 18, 2008).
278. Scrimshaw and Murray, 1988.
279. Pearson et al., 1993.
280. Andersson et al., 1984.
281. Simko and Linscheer, 1976. The elemental diets were Vivonex HN (1.9 g fat per 2,440-calorie feeding), Jejunal (2.4 g fat per 2,660-calorie feeding), and Codelid (no fat). The low-fat semi-elemental formula was Precision LR (1.9 g fat per 2,500-calorie feeding) and the higher-fat semi-elemental formula was Flexical (87 g fat per 2,612-calorie feeding).
282. Russell and Hall, 1979; Main et al., 1980; Poulin and Langevin, 1982; McIntyre et al., 1983; Heymsfield et al., 1983; Allison, 1986; Jones et al., 2004.
283. Kusumoto, 2001; Ajinomoto Co., Inc., "Encyclopedia of amino acids. 1996-2003," available at http://www.ajinomoto.com/amino/eng/product .html (accessed April 21, 2008).
284. Scheurlen et al., 1989.
285. Griffiths et al., 2000. The semi-elemental formula also included prebiotics (fructooligosaccharides); see note 288.
286. Akobeng et al., 2000.
287. Niness, 1999.
288. Griffiths et al., 2000. The formula Optimental contained fructooligosaccharides (Gloria Espinosa, Communications Coordinator, Abbott Nutrition, Public Affairs, e-mail message to the author, August 15, 2008).

289. Ste-Marie, 1982. Such a study was performed several years later (Munkholm et al., 1989) and patients seemed to respond equally well to a semi-elemental diet and a blenderized diet, but the trial was too limited to provide conclusive evidence. There were only six patients with Crohn's who completed treatment in each group, and they all began the study with normal blood work (ESR, hemoglobin, etc.) in spite of slightly or moderately active disease, so it would be difficult to tell whether either diet had an anti-inflammatory effect.
290. Korelitz, 2000.

**Chapter 8**
291. Lochs, Egger-Schödl, Pötzi, et al., 1984; Alun Jones, 1987; Greenberg et al., 1988; Wright and Adler, 1990; Furukawa et al., 1997; Kobayashi et al., 1998.
292. Stein and the German Society for Digestive and Metabolic Diseases, 2003.
293. Stokes and Irving, 1988.
294. Galandiuk et al., 1990.
295. Randall, 1990; O'Sullivan and O'Moráin, 2004.
296. O'Moráin et al., 1984; González-Huix, de Léon, et al., 1993; Seidman, Griffiths, et al., 1993.
297. Sanderson, Udeen, et al., 1987; Chafai et al., 1995; Berni Canani et al., 2006.
298. Gineston et al., 1989.
299. McCamman et al., 1977.
300. Mahajan et al., 1977; Israel and Hassall, 1995; Cosgrove and Jenkins, 1997; Anstee and Forbes, 2000.
301. Gorman et al., 2002. Another study found reductions in vitamin C and vitamin E levels in children using an enteral nutrition formula that supplied adequate quantities of those nutrients (Akobeng et al., 2007). The reason for the finding was not investigated, but if the formula was not freshly prepared before each feeding, perhaps degradation of the nutrients played a role. Selenium deficiency has also been reported, but only in patients using a formula that had no selenium in it, or one that contained less than the recommended daily allowance of selenium (Yagi et al., 1996; Kuroki et al., 2003).
302. Gavin et al., 2005.
303. Seidman, Justinich, and Roy, 1993.

304. Le Quintrec et al., 1987; Gorard et al., 1993; Teahon, Pearson, Smith, and Bjarnason, 1995.

305. Aiges et al., 1989; Israel and Hassall, 1995.

306. Werlin, 1981.

307. E.g., Ó'Moráin et al., 1984; Coyle and Sladen, 1989; Park et al., 1991; Yamamoto et al., 2005.

308. Melnik, 1990.

309. Melnik, 1990.

310. E.g., Saklad et al., 1986; Valli et al., 1986; Sneed and Morgan, 1988; Guidry et al., 1989; Melnik, 1990; O'Hagan and Wallace, 1994.

311. Melnik, 1990; Scott, 1980.

312. Gorman et al., 2002.

313. Axelsson and Jarnum, "Elemental diet in gastrointestinal diseases," 1977.

314. Silvis and Paragas, 1972; Afzal et al., 2002.

315. Silvis and Paragas, 1972.

316. Maier-Dobersberger and Lochs, 1994; Afzal et al., 2002.

317. Maier-Dobersberger and Lochs, 1994; Teahon, Pearson, Levi, and Bjarnason, 1995; Afzal et al., 2002.

318. Chiba et al., 1987; Waki et al., 1998.

319. Waki et al., 1998.

320. Berg et al., 1972; Martín Peña et al., 1990.

321. Rees et al., 1986.

322. McCamman et al., 1977.

323. Winitz, Seedman, and Graff, 1970.

324. Teahon, Pearson, Levi, and Bjarnason, 1995.

325. Fell, 2005 (see the discussion following the article).

326. Luvigsson et al., 2004.

327. Giaffer et al., 1990; Royall et al., 1994; Mansfield et al., 1995; Woolner et al., 1998.

328. Raouf et al., 1991.

329. Payne-James and Silk, 1990.

330. Griffiths, 2005 (see the discussion following the article).

331. Teahon, Pearson, Levi, and Bjarnason, 1995.

332. Johnson et al., 2006.

333. Morin et al., 1980.

334. Fell et al., 2000.

335. O'Moráin et al., 1983.

336. Thomas, Taylor, and Miller, 1993.
337. Randell and Murphy, 2001.
338. Park and Russell, 1990 (see the author reply by Giaffer and Holdsworth).
339. Zoli et al., 1997.
340. Saint-Raymond et al., 1988.
341. Oriuchi et al, 2003.

**Chapter 9**
342. Heaton et al., 1979.
343. Levenstein et al., 1985.
344. Ritchie et al., 1987.
345. E.g., Raouf et al., 1991.
346. Lorenz-Meyer et al., 1996.
347. Barclay et al., 1992.
348. Lomer et al., 2001; Lomer et al., 2004.
349. Lomer et al., 2001.
350. Lomer et al., 2005.
351. Lomer et al., 2004.
352. Maté et al., 1991.
353. Romano et al., 2005.
354. Belluzzi et al., 1996.
355. Lorenz-Meyer et al., 1996; Feagan et al., 2008.
356. Lorenz et al., 1989.
357. Belluzzi et al., 1996; Romano et al., 2005.
358. MacLean et al., 2005.
359. Holt et al., 2005.
360. Atkinson and Hunter, 2003.
361. Holt et al., 2005.
362. Juteau et al., 2003; Kordali, Cakir, et al., 2005; Kordali, Kotan, et al., 2005; Blagojević et al., 2006; Caner et al., 2008.
363. Omer et al., 2007.
364. Burkhard et al., 1999; Perazzo et al., 2003.
365. Herbs at a glance: aloe vera," National Center for Complementary and Alternative Medicine Publication No. D333, December 2006, available at http://nccam.nih.gov/health/aloevera/ (accessed July 20, 2007).
366. Alun Jones et al., 1985.
367. Alun Jones, 1987.
368. Stange et al., 1990.

369. Pearson et al., 1993.

370. Giaffer, Cann, and Holdsworth, 1991.

371. King et al., "Review article," 1997.

372. Workman et al., 1984.

373. King et al., "Review article," 1997.

374. Woolner et al., 1998.

375. Scrimshaw and Murray, 1988.

376. Park et al., 1990; Mishkin, 1994; Mishkin et al., 1997; Von Tirpitz et al., 2002.

377. von Tirpitz et al., 2002.

378. Mishkin et al., 1997.

379. Scrimshaw and Murray, 1988; Suarez et al., 1995.

380. Rowe et al., 1953; Ginsburg and Albert, "Treatment of patient with severe steroid-dependent Crohn's disease," 1989.

381. von Tirpitz et al., 2002.

382. Elsen, 2006.

383. Elsen, 2006.

384. Gionchetti et al., 2003; Mimura et al., 2004.

385. Gupta et al., 2000.

386. Prantera et al., 2002; Schultz et al., 2004; Bousvaros et al., 2005.

387. Marteau et al., 2006; Van Gossum et al., 2007.

388. Malchow, 1997.

389. Campieri et al., 2000; Guslandi et al., 2000; Karimi et al., 2005.

390. Rolfe et al., 2006.

391. Prantera et al., 2002.

392. Zunic, 1991; Riquelme et al., 2003; Kunz et al., 2004; De Groote et al., 2005.

393. Niness, 1999.

394. Lindsay et al., 2006.

395. Teramoto et al., 1996.

396. Chermesh et al., 2007.

397. D. Gordon, "The Specific Carbohydrate Diet: does it work?" Crohn's & Colitis Foundation of America, available at http://www.ccfa.org/about/news/scd (accessed July 2, 2007); Gottschall, 1994.

398. Imes et al., 1988.

399. Hilsden et al., 2003.

# GLOSSARY

**abscess** A pocket of pus, usually caused by an infection, or more rarely by an irritant such as an injected drug.

**alpha-4 integrin** A protein that plays a role in the body's inflammatory process.

**amino acids** Small molecules that are the building blocks of protein. Used in elemental and some semi-elemental formulas as ingredients from which our bodies can synthesize protein.

**aminosalicylates** Mild anti-inflammatory medications such as sulfasalazine and mesalamine; used for people with IBD.

**anabolic steroids** Synthetic versions of male sex hormones; sometimes abused by athletes or weightlifters. Different from the corticosteroids often used by people with Crohn's.

**anus** The opening through which stool leaves the body.

**aphthous ulcers** Sores inside the mouth, on the gums, or the tongue.

**arthralgias** Joint pains without visible inflammation.

**arthritis** Joint pain accompanied by swelling and stiffness.

**biologics**  Drugs such as Remicade and Humira  that are made from living organisms or their products.

**biopsies**  Small samples of tissue taken from the body and examined under a microscope.

**bolus feeding**  Method of tube feeding in which enteral nutrition is given as "meals" several times per day rather than continuously throughout the day.

**brand name**  The name assigned to a drug for marketing purposes. A single drug may have more than one brand name. Brand names are usually capitalized. Compare *generic name*.


**catch-up growth**  Faster than normal growth in children who previously had growth delays, allowing them to "catch up" on some or all of the growth they missed.

**celiac disease**  Disease caused by an inability to digest gluten, a protein found in many grains.

**continuous-drip feeding**  Method of tube feeding in which the formula is dripped continuously through a tube throughout the day or night or both.

**colectomy**  Surgical removal of all or part of the colon.

**colon**  The longest portion of the large intestine; made up of the ascending colon, transverse colon, descending colon, and sigmoid colon.

**colostomy**  Surgery to connect the colon to an opening created in the abdomen for the excretion of wastes; allows removal or bypassing of the rectum. The term "colostomy" is also used to refer to the opening that is created by the surgery.

**corticosteroids**  Class of medications with a powerful anti-inflammatory effect. Can also be referred to as glucocorticoids or steroids.

**C-reactive protein** A protein produced by the liver and released into the bloodstream. Elevated levels are a sign of inflammation somewhere in the body.

**Crohn's colitis** Crohn's disease affecting the large intestine but not other parts of the gastrointestinal tract.

**Crohn's disease** An inflammatory bowel disease in which areas of inflammation can occur anywhere in the gastrointestinal tract from the mouth to the anus.

**duodenum** The first of the three sections of the small intestine.

**electrolytes** Substances (mainly minerals) present in body fluids that have positive or negative electric charges and help regulate bodily functions.

**elemental formulas** Enteral nutrition formulas that supply protein in the form of amino acids. Also called elemental diets.

**endoscope** Tube with a tiny camera attached to the end used to look inside the gastrointestinal tract. Inserted through the mouth to examine the stomach, esophagus, and upper part of the small intestine or through the anus to examine the large intestine.

**endoscopic balloon dilation** Using an endoscope to insert a small balloon or dilator into a stricture and then widening the stricture by inflating and deflating the balloon or inserting successively larger dilators.

**endoscopic improvement** Healing of the intestines as assessed through an endoscope.

**endoscopic recurrence** Recurrence of damage to the intestines that can be seen through an endoscope.

**endoscopy** Procedure in which a doctor uses a tube with a tiny camera at the end to look at the insides of the small intestine and take biopsies.

**enteral nutrition**  Liquid diets used in place of, or in addition to, normal food.

**episcleritis**  Inflammation of the membrane (episclera) that covers the white part of the eye. Can be a complication of Crohn's.

**erythrocyte sedimentation rate**  Test that measures how many erythrocytes (red blood cells) settle to the bottom of a test tube within one hour. Also referred to as ESR or sed rate. A raised erythrocyte sedimentation rate is a sign of inflammation.

**esophagus**  The tube connecting the mouth with the stomach.

**ESR**  Abbreviation for erythrocyte sedimentation rate.

**extraintestinal symptom**  Complication of Crohn's disease affecting an organ or area of the body outside the gastrointestinal tract.

**fissure**  Tear in the skin.

**fistula**  Abnormal passage that opens up between two areas of the body that would not normally be connected, such as the colon and the bladder (colovesical fistula) or the vagina and rectum (rectovaginal fistula).

**flare**  Occurrence or recurrence of active disease.

**food allergy**  Immunological reaction to a protein found in food. Can cause symptoms throughout the body, not just digestive symptoms.

**food intolerance**  A reaction to a food that affects the digestive system only (e.g., diarrhea or bloating) and not the immune system.

**gastrostomy**  Artificially created opening in the abdomen to which a feeding tube can be connected to deliver enteral nutrition directly to the stomach.

**generic name**  A drug's official name. Usually generic names are not capitalized. Compare *brand name*.

**growth failure**  Slower than normal growth in children or cessation of growth.

**hemicolectomy**  Surgery to remove a portion of the colon.

**histologic improvement**  Healing of the intestines as assessed by examining samples of intestinal tissue under a microscope.

**histologic recurrence**  Recurrence of damage to the intestines that may not be visible to the eye but is apparent when examining a tissue sample under a microscope.

**hydrolyzed protein**  Whole protein that has been broken down by the addition of water into smaller molecules called peptides. Less likely to cause allergic reactions in people with food allergies than whole protein.

**IBD**  Abbreviation for inflammatory bowel disease.

**IBS**  Abbreviation for irritable bowel syndrome.

**ileocolonic**  Relating to both the ileum and the colon.

**ileostomy**  Surgery to connect the ileum to an opening created in the abdomen for the excretion of wastes; allows removal or bypassing of the colon and/or rectum. The term "ileostomy" is also used to refer to the opening created in the abdomen.

**ileum**  The third and last section of the small intestine.

**immunomodulators**  Medications such as 6-MP, azathiaprine, and methotrexate that are designed to reduce the activity of an overactive immune system to more normal levels. Also referred to as immunosuppressives.

**indeterminate colitis**  Inflammatory bowel disease that resembles Crohn's disease and ulcerative colitis but is not clearly diagnosable as one or the other.

**inflammatory bowel disease**  Any of a number of chronic diseases that cause inflammation in the intestines, including Crohn's disease, ulcerative colitis, indeterminate colitis, collagenous colitis, lymphocytic colitis, and others. Abbreviated as IBD.

**intestinal mucosa** The layer of tissue forming the inner walls of the intestines.

**irritable bowel syndrome** Condition characterized by gastro-intestinal symptoms such as constipation, diarrhea, pain, and/or bloating without physical signs of disease such as inflammation or bleeding.

**jejunostomy** Surgery to create an opening from the abdominal wall to the jejunum to allow insertion of a feeding tube or for the excretion of wastes. The term "jejunostomy" is also used to refer to the opening that is created by the surgery.

**jejunum** The second of the three sections of the small intestine.

**lactase** Enzyme in the small intestine that breaks down lactose into easily digested simple sugars.

**lactose** Milk sugar (the carbohydrate found in milk).

**large intestine** The section of the gastrointestinal tract con-necting the small intestine with the anus. Made up of the cecum, appendix, ascending colon, transverse colon, descending colon, sigmoid colon, and rectum.

**maintenance therapy** In people with IBD, any treatment used on a long-term basis to maintain remission.

**monomeric diets** Another way of referring to elemental enteral nutrition formulas.

**mucosal healing** Healing of the tissue called the mucosa that lines the gastrointestinal tract.

**nasoduodenal tube** Feeding tube inserted through the nose and ending in the duodenum, the first section of the small intestine.

**nasogastric tube** Feeding tube inserted through the nose and ending in the stomach.

**nasojejunal tube** Feeding tube inserted through the nose and ending in the jejunum, the second section of the small intestine.

**oligomeric diets**  Another way of referring to semi-elemental enteral nutrition formulas.

**oligopeptide diets**  Yet another way of referring to semi-elemental formulas.

**osmolality**  The concentration of particles in a fluid.

**osteopenia**  Low bone density; the forerunner of osteoporosis.

**osteoporosis**  Disease causing brittle, porous bones that can break easily.

**ostomy**  Surgery to create an opening (stoma) in the skin of the abdomen for the excretion of wastes.

**parenteral nutrition**  Liquid food delivered straight into the bloodstream through a small tube inserted into a vein. Also called intravenous feeding

**peptides**  Small to medium-sized molecules made up of amino acids linked together in short chains. The sole or main source of protein in semi-elemental formulas.

**perianal disease**  Crohn's symptoms affecting the anal and perineal area, most commonly fissures, fistulas, and ulcers.

**placebo**  A substance that resembles a medication but doesn't have any disease-fighting activity.

**placebo-controlled study**  A study in which patients are randomly assigned to receive a placebo or a medical treatment in order to find out whether the treatment is more effective than a placebo.

**polymeric formulas**  Enteral nutrition formulas containing whole protein. Also called polymeric diets.

**prebiotics**  Term used to refer to some types of plant fiber (most commonly the fructooligosaccharides inulin and oligofructose) that may be added to food and beverages to increase their fiber content.

**probiotics**  Microorganisms that may be beneficial to their hosts and do not normally cause disease.

**prospective study**  A study of a medical treatment in which the patients are given a treatment and then observed to see whether they respond to it. The dose and duration of the treatment and the criteria used to determine whether someone has responded to it are decided in advance.

**proctocolectomy**  Surgery to remove the rectum and all or part of the colon.

**randomized study**  A prospective study in which patients are randomly assigned to the treatments being tested. See *prospective study.*

**rectum**  The last part of the large intestine; the place where stool is stored until excretion.

**refeeding syndrome**  Potentially serious disturbance in the body's balance of fluids and electrolytes.

**relapse**  Reoccurrence of disease symptoms after a period of remission. See *remission.*

**remission**  Period of time during which disease is inactive (minimal or no symptoms, normal or near-normal blood work). Remissions can be brief or can last for months or years.

**resection**  Surgery to remove a diseased or strictured area of intestine.

**retrospective study**  A medical study performed by analyzing data collected from the records of patients who have already received a given treatment.

**scleritis**  Inflammation of the white of the eye (the sclera). Can be a complication of Crohn's.

**semi-elemental formulas**  Enteral nutrition formulas that supply protein in the form of peptides or as a mix of amino acids and peptides. Also called semi-elemental diets.

**short-bowel syndrome** Poor absorption of food due to removal of a large portion of the small intestine, often resulting in diarrhea, dehydration, and malnutrition.

**small bowel** Another name for the small intestine.

**small intestine** The part of the gastrointestinal tract connecting the stomach and the large intestine. It has three parts: the duodenum, jejunum, and ileum.

**stenosis** Narrowed area of intestine that can make it difficult for food to pass through. Also referred to as a stricture.

**steroid-dependent** Unable to remain in remission if steroids are discontinued.

**steroid-refractory** Fails to go into remission when given steroids.

**steroids** Abbreviation for corticosteroids, powerful anti-inflammatory drugs. Sometimes also used as an abbreviation for anabolic steroids.

**stoma** Artificial opening in the skin of the abdomen created surgically to allow the excretion of wastes.

**stricture** Narrowed area of intestine that can make it difficult for food to pass through. Also referred to as a stenosis.

**stricturoplasty** Surgical procedure in which a narrowed area of intestine is incised lengthwise and sewed back together crosswise in order to widen rather than remove a strictured area.

**supplemental enteral nutrition** Enteral nutrition used in addition to normal food to supply a portion of a person's daily nutritional needs.

**synbiotic** Product containing both probiotics and prebiotics.

**terminal ileum** The very end of the ileum; see *ileum*.
**TNF-α** Abbreviation for tumor necrosis factor-α, a protein made by the immune system that causes inflammation.

**total enteral nutrition** Enteral nutrition used instead of normal food to supply all of a person's nutritional needs.

**total parenteral nutrition** Parenteral nutrition used instead of normal food to supply all of a person's nutritional needs. Commonly referred to as TPN. See *parenteral nutrition.*

**TPN** Abbreviation for total parental nutrition.

**tumor necrosis factor-α** Protein made by the immune system that causes inflammation. Often abbreviated as TNF-α.

**ulcerative colitis** An inflammatory bowel disease in which inflammation affects the inner lining of the large intestine but not other parts of the gastrointestinal tract.

**uveitis** Inflammation of the lining of the eyeball (the uvea). Can be a complication of Crohn's.

# BIBLIOGRAPHY

Abad-Lacruz A, González-Huix F, Esteve M, et al. Liver function tests [sic] abnormalities in patients with inflammatory bowel disease receiving artificial nutrition: a prospective randomized study of total enteral nutrition vs total parenteral nutrition. *JPEN J Parenter Enteral Nutr*. 1990 Nov-Dec;14(6):618-21.

Afdhal NH, Kelly J, McCormick PA, O'Donoghue DP. Remission induction in refractory Crohn's disease using a high calorie whole diet. *JPEN J Parenter Enteral Nutr*. 1989 Jul-Aug;13(4):362-5.

Afzal NA, Addai S, Fagbemi A, Murch S, Thomson M, Heuschkel R. Refeeding syndrome with enteral nutrition in children: a case report, literature review and clinical guidelines. *Clin Nutr*. 2002 Dec;21(6): 515-20.

Afzal NA, Davies S, Paintin M, et al. Colonic Crohn's disease in children does not respond well to treatment with enteral nutrition if the ileum is not involved. *Dig Dis Sci*. 2005 Aug;50(8):1471-5.

Afzal NA, Van Der Zaag-Loonen HJ, Arnaud-Battandier F, et al. Improvement in quality of life of children with acute Crohn's disease does not parallel mucosal healing after treatment with exclusive enteral nutrition. *Aliment Pharmacol Ther*. 2004 Jul 15;20(2):167-72.

Aiges H, Markowitz J, Rosa J, Daum F. Home nocturnal supplemental nasogastric feedings in growth-retarded adolescents with Crohn's disease. *Gastroenterology*. 1989 Oct;97(4):905-10.

Akobeng AI, Clayton PE, Miller V, Hall CM, Thomas AG. Low serum concentrations of insulin-like growth factor-I in children with active Crohn disease: effect of enteral nutritional support and glutamine supplementation. *Scand J Gastroenterol.* 2002 Dec;37(12):1422-7.

Akobeng AK, Miller V, Stanton J, Elbadri AM, Thomas AG. Double-blind randomized controlled trial of glutamine-enriched polymeric diet in the treatment of active Crohn's disease. *J Pediatr Gastroenterol Nutr.* 2000 Jan;30(1):78-84.

Akobeng AK, Richmond K, Miller V, Thomas AG. Effect of exclusive enteral nutritional treatment on plasma antioxidant concentrations in childhood Crohn's disease. *Clin Nutr.* 2007;26:51-6.

Akobeng AK, Thomas AG. Enteral nutrition for maintenance of remission in Crohn's disease. *Cochrane Database Syst Rev.* 2007 Jul 18;(3):CD005984.

Akobeng AK, Richmond K, Miller V, Thomas AG. Effect of exclusive enteral nutritional treatment on plasma antioxidant concentrations in childhood Crohn's disease. *Clin Nutr.* 2007 Feb;26(1):51-6. Epub 2006 Dec 11

Allison SP. Some psychological and physiological aspects of enteral nutrition. *Gut.* 1986 Nov;27 Suppl 1:18-24.

Alun Jones V. Comparison of total parenteral nutrition and elemental diet in induction of remission of Crohn's disease. Long-term maintenance of remission by personalized food exclusion diets. *Dig Dis Sci.* 1987 Dec;32(12 Suppl):100S-107S.

Alun Jones V, Dickinson RJ, Workman E, Wilson AJ, Freeman AH, Hunter JO. Crohn's disease: maintenance of remission by diet. *Lancet.* 1985 Jul 27;2(8448):177-80.

Andersson H, Bosaeus I, Ellegard L, Hallgren B, Hultén L, Magnusson O. Comparison of an elemental and two polymeric diets in colectomized patients with or without intestinal resection. *Clin Nutr.* 1984 Dec;3(4):183-9.

Anstee QM, Forbes A. The safe use of percutaneous gastrostomy for enteral nutrition in patients with Crohn's disease. *Eur J Gastroenterol Hepatol.* 2000 Oct;12(10):1089-93.

Arber N, Odes HS, Fireman Z, et al. A controlled double blind multicenter study of the effectiveness of 5-aminosalicylic acid in patients with Crohn's disease in remission. *J Clin Gastroenterol.* 1995 Apr;20(3):203-6.

Ardizzone S, Bollani S, Manzionna G, Imbesi V, Colombo E, Bianchi Porro G. Comparison between methotrexate and azathioprine in the treatment of chronic active Crohn's disease: a randomised, investigator-blind study. *Dig Liver Dis.* 2003 Sep;35(9):619-27.

Ardizzone S, Colombo E, Maconi G, et al. Infliximab in treatment of Crohn's disease: the Milan experience. *Dig Liver Dis.* 2002 Jun;34(6):411-8.

Ardizzone S, Maconi G, Colombo E, Manzionna G, Bollani S, Bianchi Porro G. Perianal fistulae following infliximab treatment: clinical and endosonographic outcome. *Inflamm Bowel Dis.* 2004 Mar;10(2):91-6.

Arnold GL, Beaves MR, Pryjdun VO, Mook WJ. Preliminary study of ciprofloxacin in active Crohn's disease. *Inflamm Bowel Dis.* 2002 Jan;8(1):10-5.

Arnott IDR, Ghosh S, Drummond HE, Ferguson A, Maguire C, Russell RCG. Improvement in whole gut lavage fluid inflammatory markers in patients with Crohn's disease treated with elemental diet [abstract P827]. *Gut.* 1997; 41 Suppl 3:A225.

Arora S, Katkov W, Cooley J, et al. Methotrexate in Crohn's disease: results of a randomized, double-blind, placebo-controlled trial. *Hepatogastroenterology.* 1999 May-Jun;46(27):1724-9.

Atkinson RJ, Hunter JO. A double blind, placebo controlled randomised trial of Curcuma extract in the treatment of steroid dependent inflammatory bowel disease [abstract S1377]. *Gastroenterology.* 2003 Apr; 124 Suppl 1:A-205.

Axelsson C, Jarnum S. Assessment of the therapeutic value of an elemental diet in chronic inflammatory bowel disease. *Scand J Gastroenterol.* 1977;12(1):89-95.

Axelsson C, Jarnum S. Elemental diet in gastrointestinal diseases: experience from a case material of 59 patients. *Infusionsther Klin Ernahr.* 1977 Dec;4(6):313-8.

Axelsson CK, Jarnum S. Influence of an elemental diet in protein exudation in chronic inflammatory bowel disease. *Digestion.* 1977;16(1-2):77-86.

Axelsson CK, Justesen T. Studies of the duodenal and fecal flora in gastrointestinal disorders during treatment with an elemental diet. Gastroenterology. 1977 Mar;72(3):397-401.

Azcue M, Rashid M, Griffiths A, Pencharz PB. Energy expenditure and body composition in children with Crohn's disease: effect of enteral nutrition and treatment with prednisolone. *Gut.* 1997 Aug;41(2):203-8.

Baba S, Nakai K. Strictureplasty for Crohn's disease in Japan. *J Gastroenterol.* 1995 Nov;30 Suppl 8:135-8.

Bamba T, Shimoyama T, Sasaki M, et al. Dietary fat attenuates the benefits of an elemental diet in active Crohn's disease: a randomized, controlled trial. *Eur J Gastroenterol Hepatol.* 2003 Feb;15(2):151-7.

Bannerjee K, Camacho-Hübner C, Babinska K, et al. Anti-inflammatory and growth-stimulating effects precede nutritional restitution during enteral feeding in Crohn disease. *J Pediatr Gastroenterol Nutr*. 2004 Mar;38(3):270-5.

Barclay GR, McKenzie H, Pennington J, Parratt D, Pennington CR. The effect of dietary yeast on the activity of stable chronic Crohn's disease. *Scand J Gastroenterol*. 1992;27(3):196-200.

Bar-Meir S, Chowers Y, Lavy A, et al. Budesonide versus prednisone in the treatment of active Crohn's disease. The Israeli Budesonide Study Group. *Gastroenterology*. 1998 Oct;115(4):835-40.

Beattie RM. Enteral nutrition as primary therapy in childhood Crohn's disease: control of intestinal inflammation and anabolic response. *JPEN J Parenter Enteral Nutr*. 2005 Jul-Aug;29(4 Suppl):S151-5; discussion S155-9, S184-8.

Beattie RM, Camacho-Hübner C, Wacharasindhu S, Cotterill AM, Walker-Smith JA, Savage MO. Responsiveness of IGF-I and IGFBP-3 to therapeutic intervention in children and adolescents with Crohn's disease. *Clin Endocrinol (Oxf)*. 1998 Oct;49(4):483-9.

Beattie RM. Nutritional management of Crohn's disease in childhood. *J R Soc Med*. 1998 Mar;91(3):135-7.

Beattie RM, Schiffrin EJ, Donnet-Hughes A, et al. Polymeric nutrition as the primary therapy in children with small bowel Crohn's disease. *Aliment Pharmacol Ther*. 1994 Dec;8(6):609-15.

Belli DC, Seidman E, Bouthillier L, et al. Chronic intermittent elemental diet improves growth failure in children with Crohn's disease. *Gastroenterology*. 1988 Mar;94(3):603-10.

Belluzzi A, Brignola C, Campieri M, Pera A, Boschi S, Miglioli M. Effect of an enteric-coated fish-oil preparation on relapses in Crohn's disease. *N Engl J Med*. 1996 Jun 13;334(24):1557-60.

Berg G, Classen M. Experience with balanced, bulk-free nutrition in Crohn's disease and ulcerative colitis [in German]. *Med Klin*. 1973 Apr 13;68(15):487-90.

Berg G, Wagner H, Weber L. Balanced residue-free diet in intestinal diseases [in German]. *Dtsch Med Wochenschr*. 1972 May 26;97(21):826-9 passim.

Berni Canani R, Terrin G, et al. Short- and long-term therapeutic efficacy of nutritional therapy and corticosteroids in paediatric Crohn's disease. *Dig Liver Dis*. 2006 Jun;38(6):381-7. Epub 2005 Nov 18.

Bernstein CN, Shanahan F. Braving the elementals in Crohn's disease. *Gastroenterology*. 1992 Oct;103(4):1363-4.

Bernstein LH, Frank MS, Brandt LJ, Boley SJ. Healing of perineal Crohn's disease with metronidazole. *Gastroenterology.* 1980 Sep;79(3):599.

Blackburn GL, Bell ST, Georgieff M. Enteral tube feeding: state of the art. *Z Gastroenterol.* 1985 Aug;23 Suppl:7-15.

Blagojević P, Radulović N, Palić R, Stojanović G. Chemical composition of the essential oils of serbian wild-growing *Artemisia absinthium* and *Artemisia vulgaris. J Agric Food Chem.* 2006 Jun 28;54(13):4780-9.

Blair GK, Yaman M, Wesson DE. Preoperative home elemental enteral nutrition in complicated Crohn's disease. *J Pediatr Surg.* 1986 Sep;21(9): 769-71.

Bodemar G, Nilsson L, Smedh K, Larsson J. Nasogastric feeding with polymeric, whole protein, low fat diet in Crohn's disease. *J Clin Gastroenterol.* 1991 Apr-Jun;6(2):75-83.

Borrelli O, Bascietto C, Viola F, et al. Infliximab heals intestinal inflammatory lesions and restores growth in children with Crohn's disease. *Dig Liver Dis.* 2004 May;36(5):342-7.

Borrelli O, Cordischi L, Cirulli M, et al. Polymeric diet alone versus corticosteroids in the treatment of active pediatric Crohn's disease: a randomized controlled open-label trial. *Clin Gastroenterol Hepatol.* 2006 Jun;4(6): 744-53. Epub 2006 May 6.

Bounous G, Devroede G, Haddad H, Beaudry R, Perey BJ, Lejeune LP. Use of an elemental diet for intestinal disorders and for the critically ill. *Dis Colon Rectum.* 1974 Mar-Apr;17(2):157-65.

Bousvaros A, Guandalini S, Baldassano RN, et al. A randomized, double-blind trial of *Lactobacillus* GG versus placebo in addition to standard maintenance therapy for children with Crohn's disease. *Inflamm Bowel Dis.* 2005 Sep;11(9):833-9.

Brandt LJ, Bernstein LH, Boley SJ, Frank MS. Metronidazole therapy for perineal Crohn's disease: a follow-up study. *Gastroenterology.* 1982 Aug;83(2):383-7.

Breese EJ, Michie CA, Nicholls SW, et al. The effect of treatment on lymphokine-secreting cells in the intestinal mucosa of children with Crohn's disease. *Aliment Pharmacol Ther.* 1995 Oct;9(5):547-52.

Breese EJ, Michie CA, Nicholls SW, et al. Tumor necrosis factor alpha-producing cells in the intestinal mucosa of children with inflammatory bowel disease. *Gastroenterology.* 1994 Jun;106(6):1455-66.

Bret M, Souquet JC. Exclusive semi-elemental enteral nutrition in Crohn's disease [in French]. *Gastroenterol Clin Biol.* 1988 May;12(5):501.

Brignola C, Cottone M, Pera A, et al. Mesalamine in the prevention of endo-scopic recurrence after intestinal resection for Crohn's disease. Italian Cooperative Study Group. *Gastroenterology*. 1995 Feb;108(2):345-9.

Brignola C, Iannone P, Pasquali S, et al. Placebo-controlled trial of oral 5-ASA in relapse prevention of Crohn's disease. *Dig Dis Sci*. 1992 Jan;37(1):29-32.

Brignola C, Lanfranchi GA, Pasquali R, Campieri M, Bazzocchi G, Veggetti S. Calorie supplementation and Crohn's disease. *Lancet*. 1983 Jul 2;2(8340): 47.

Burgmann T, Clara I, Graff L, et al. The Manitoba Inflammatory Bowel Dis-ease Cohort Study: prolonged symptoms before diagnosis—how much is irritable bowel syndrome? *Clin Gastroenterol Hepatol*. 2006 May;4(5): 614-20. Epub 2006 Apr 17.

Burkhard PR, Burkhardt K, Haenggeli CA, Landis T. Plant-induced seizures: reappearance of an old problem. *J Neurol*. 1999 Aug;246(8):667-70.

Bury KD, Stephens RV, Randall HT. Use of a chemically defined, liquid, elemental diet for nutritional management of fistulas of the alimentary tract. *Am J Surg*. 1971 Feb;121(2):174-83.


Calam J, Crooks PE, Walker RJ. Elemental diets in the management of Crohn's perianal fistulae. *JPEN J Parenter Enteral Nutr*. 1980 Jan-Feb;4(1):4-8.

Cameron EA, Middleton SJ. Elemental diet in the treatment of orofacial Crohn's disease. *Gut*. 2003 Jan;52(1):143.

Campieri M, Ferguson A, Doe W, Persson T, Nilsson LG. Oral budesonide is as effective as oral prednisolone in active Crohn's disease. The Global Budesonide Study Group. *Gut*. 1997 Aug;41(2):209-14.

Campieri M, Rizzello E, Venturi A, et al. Combination of antibiotic and probiotic treatment is efficacious in prophylaxis of post-operative recurrence of Crohn's disease: a randomized, controlled study vs. mesalamine [abstract 4179]. *Gastroenterology*. 2000 Apr;118(4):A781.

Candy S, Wright J, Gerber M, Adams G, Gerig M, Goodman R. A controlled double blind study of azathioprine in the management of Crohn's disease. *Gut*. 1995 Nov;37(5):674-8.

Caner A, Döşkaya M, Değirmenci A, et al. Comparison of the effects of *Artemisia vulgaris* and *Artemisia absinthium* growing in western Anatolia against trichinellosis (*Trichinella spiralis*) in rats. *Exp Parasitol*. 2008 May;119(1):173-9. Epub 2008 Feb 5.

Capristo E, Mingrone G, Addolorato G, Greco AV, Gasbarrini G. Effect of a vegetable-protein-rich polymeric diet treatment on body composition and energy metabolism in inactive Crohn's disease. *Eur J Gastroenterol Hepatol.* 2000 Jan;12(1):5-11.

Carter MJ, Lobo AJ, Travis SP; IBD Section, British Society of Gastroenterology. Guidelines for the management of inflammatory bowel disease in adults. *Gut.* 2004 Sep;53 Suppl 5:V1-16.

Cezard JP, Messing B. Enteral nutrition in inflammatory bowel diseases: is there a special role for elemental diets? *Clin Nutr.* 1993;12(Suppl 1): S75-S81.

Cezard JP, Nouaili N, Talbotec C, et al. A prospective study of the efficacy and tolerance of a chimeric antibody to tumor necrosis factors (Remicade) in severe pediatric Crohn's disease. *J Pediatr Gastroenterol Nutr.* 2003 May;36(5):632-6.

Chafai S, Martin D, Goulet O, Mougenot JF, Ricour C, Schmitz J. Semi-elemental diet and corticosteroids in the treatment of Crohn's disease in children [abstract 82]. *J Pediatr Gastroenterol Nutr.* 1995;20(4):465.

Chebli JM, Gaburri PD, De Souza AF, et al. Long-term results with azathioprine therapy in patients with corticosteroid-dependent Crohn's disease: open-label prospective study. *J Gastroenterol Hepatol.* 2007 Feb;22(2): 268-74.

Chermesh I, Tamir A, Reshef R, et al. Failure of Synbiotic 2000 to prevent postoperative recurrence of Crohn's disease. *Dig Dis Sci.* 2007 Feb;52(2): 385-9. Epub 2007 Jan 9.

Chiba M, Igarashi K, Ohta H, Ohtaka M, Arakawa H, Masamune O. Rhabdomyolysis associated with Crohn's disease. *Jpn J Med.* 1987 May;26(2): 255-60.

Chong RY, Hanauer SB, Cohen RD. Efficacy of parenteral methotrexate in refractory Crohn's disease. *Aliment Pharmacol Ther.* 2001 Jan;15(1):35-44.

Collins EN, Pritchett CP. Allergy as a factor in disturbances of the gastrointestinal tract. *Med Clinics North Am.* 1938 Mar;22(2):297-317.

Colombel JF, Lémann M, Cassagnou M, et al. A controlled trial comparing ciprofloxacin with mesalazine for the treatment of active Crohn's disease. Groupe d'Etudes Thérapeutiques des Affections Inflammatoires Digestives (GETAID). *Am J Gastroenterol.* 1999 Mar;94(3):674-8.

Colombel JF, Sandborn WJ, Rutgeerts P, et al. Adalimumab for maintenance of clinical response and remission in patients with Crohn's disease: the CHARM trial. *Gastroenterology.* 2007 Jan;132(1):52-65. Epub 2006 Nov 29.

Comité de nutrition de la Société française de pédiatrie. Nutritional treatment in childhood Crohn's disease [in French]. *Arch Pediatr.* 2005 Aug;12(8):1255-66.

Cosgrove M, Jenkins HR. Experience of percutaneous endoscopic gastrostomy in children with Crohn's disease. *Arch Dis Child*. 1997 Feb;76(2):141-3.

Cosnes J, Bellanger J, Gendre JP, Le Quintrec Y. Crohn's disease and enteral feeding: comparative nutritional efficacy of elemental and polymeric nutritive mixtures [in French]. *Ann Gastroenterol Hepatol (Paris)*. 1988 Oct;24(5):233-40.

Couch RB, Watkin DM, Smith RR, et al. Clinical trials of water-soluble chemically defined diets [abstract]. *Fed Proc*. 1960;19:13.

Coyle BL, Sladen GP. Whole protein liquid diet in the treatment of acute uncomplicated Crohn's disease. *J Hum Nutr Diet*. 1989;2:25-30.

Cucchiara S, Guandalini S, Staiano A, et al. Remission of colonic Crohn's disease induced by elemental diet. *Ital J Gastroenterol*. 1984;16:302-4.

Davison SM, Johnson T, Chapman S, Booth IW, Murphy MS. Disease location in elemental diet therapy of Crohn's disease: a study of response using [99M]TC-HMPAO leukocyte scintigraphy [abstract]. *Gastroenterology*. 1996 Apr;110(4):A797.

Day AS, Whitten KE, Lemberg DA, et al. Exclusive enteral feeding as primary therapy for Crohn's disease in Australian children and adolescents: a feasible and effective approach. *J Gastroenterol Hepatol*. 2006 Oct;21(10):1609-14.

de Franchis R, Omodei P, Ranzi T, et al. Controlled trial of oral 5-aminosalicylic acid for the prevention of early relapse in Crohn's disease. *Aliment Pharmacol Ther*. 1997 Oct;11(5):845-52.

De Groote MA, Frank DN, Dowell E, Glode MP, Pace NR. *Lactobacillus rhamnosus* GG bacteremia associated with probiotic use in a child with short gut syndrome. *Pediatr Infect Dis J*. 2005 Mar;24(3):278-80.

de Jong NSH, Leach ST, Day AS. Polymeric formula has direct anti-inflammatory effects on enterocytes in an *in vitro* model of intestinal inflammation. *Dig Dis Sci*. 2007 Sep;52(9):2029-36. Epub 2007 Apr 4.

D'Haens G, Geboes K, Rutgeerts P. Endoscopic and histologic healing of Crohn's (ileo-) colitis with azathioprine. *Gastrointest Endosc*. 1999 Nov;50(5):667-71.

Dickman MD, Chappelka AR, Schaedler RW. Evaluation of gut microflora during administration of an elemental diet in a patient with an ileoproctostomy. *Dig Dis*. 1975 Apr;20(4):377-80.

Dolz C, Xiol X, Abad A, et al. Changes in liver function tests in patients with inflammatory bowel disease on enteral nutrition. *JPEN J Parenter Enteral Nutr*. 1989 Jul-Aug;13(4):401-5.

Domènech E, Hinojosa J, Nos P, et al. Clinical evolution of luminal and perianal Crohn's disease after inducing remission with infliximab: how long should patients be treated? *Aliment Pharmacol Ther.* 2005 Dec;22 (11-12):1107-13.

Dray X, Marteau P. The use of enteral nutrition in the management of Crohn's disease in adults. *JPEN J Parenter Enteral Nutr.* 2005 Jul-Aug;29(4 Suppl):S166-9; discussion S169-72, S184-8.

Driscoll RH Jr, Rosenberg IH. Total parenteral nutrition in inflammatory bowel disease. *Med Clin North Am.* 1978 Jan;62(1):185-201.

Dziechciarz P, Horvath A, Shamir R, Szajewska H. Meta-analysis: enteral nutrition in active Crohn's disease in children. *Aliment Pharmacol Ther.* 2007 Sep 15;26(6):795-806.

Elsen CO. From cheese to pharma: a designer probiotic for IBD. *Clin Gastroenterol Hepatol.* 2006 Jul;4(7):836-7.

Esaki M, Matsumoto T, Hizawa K, et al. Preventive effect of nutritional therapy against postoperative recurrence of Crohn disease, with reference to findings determined by intra-operative enteroscopy. *Scand J Gastroenterol.* 2005 Dec;40(12):1431-7.

Esaki M, Matsumoto T, Nakamura S, et al. Factors affecting recurrence in patients with Crohn's disease under nutritional therapy. *Dis Colon Rectum.* 2006 Oct;49(10 Suppl):S68-74.

Escher JC. Nutritional therapy in paediatric Crohn's disease: More food for thought? *Dig Liver Dis.* 2006 Jun;38(6):387-8. Epub 2006 Mar 29.

Escher JC, European Collaborative Research Group on Budesonide in Paediatric IBD. Budesonide versus prednisolone for the treatment of active Crohn's disease in children: a randomized, double-blind, controlled, multicentre trial. *Eur J Gastroenterol Hepatol.* 2004 Jan;16(1):47-54.

Ewe K, Böttger T, Buhr HJ, Ecker KW, Otto HF. Low-dose budesonide treatment for prevention of postoperative recurrence of Crohn's disease: a multicentre randomized placebo-controlled trial. German Budesonide Study Group. *Eur J Gastroenterol Hepatol.* 1999 Mar;11(3):277-82.

Ewe K, Herfarth C, Malchow H, Jesdinsky HJ. Postoperative recurrence of Crohn's disease in relation to radicality of operation and sulfasalazine prophylaxis: a multicenter trial. *Digestion.* 1989;42(4):224-32.

Faubion WA Jr, Loftus EV Jr, Harmsen WS, Zinsmeister AR, Sandborn WJ. The natural history of corticosteroid therapy for inflammatory bowel disease: a population-based study. *Gastroenterology.* 2001 Aug;121(2):255-60.

Feagan BG, Fedorak RN, Irvine EJ, et al. A comparison of methotrexate with placebo for the maintenance of remission in Crohn's disease. North American Crohn's Study Group Investigators. *N Engl J Med.* 2000 Jun 1;342(22):1627-32.

Feagan BG, Rochon J, Fedorak RN, et al. Methotrexate for the treatment of Crohn's disease. The North American Crohn's Study Group Investigators. *N Engl J Med.* 1995 Feb 2;332(5):292-7.

Feagan BG, Sandborn WJ, Mittmann U, et al. Omega-3 free fatty acids for the maintenance of remission in Crohn disease: the EPIC randomized controlled trials. *JAMA.* 2008 Apr 9;299(14):1690-7.

Fell JM. Control of systemic and local inflammation with transforming growth factor beta containing formulas. *JPEN J Parenter Enteral Nutr.* 2005 Jul-Aug;29(4 Suppl):S126-8; discussion S129-33, S184-8.

Fell JM, Paintin M, Arnaud-Battandier F, et al. Mucosal healing and a fall in mucosal pro-inflammatory cytokine mRNA induced by a specific oral polymeric diet in paediatric Crohn's disease. *Aliment Pharmacol Ther.* 2000 Mar;14(3):281-9.

Fell JM, Paintin M, Donnet-Hughes A, Arnaud-Battandier F, MacDonald TT, Walker-Smith JA. Remission induced by a new specific oral polymeric diet in children with Crohn's disease. *Nestle Nutr Workshop Ser Clin Perform Programme.* 1999;2:187-96; discussion 196-8.

Ferguson A, Campieri M, Doe W, Persson T, Nygård G. Oral budesonide as maintenance therapy in Crohn's disease—results of a 12-month study. Global Budesonide Study Group. *Aliment Pharmacol Ther.* 1998 Feb;12(2):175-83.

Ferguson A, Glen M, Ghosh S. Crohn's disease: nutrition and nutritional therapy. *Baillieres Clin Gastroenterol.* 1998 Mar;12(1):93-114.

Fernández-Banares F, Cabré E, Esteve-Comas M, Gassull MA. How effective is enteral nutrition in inducing clinical remission in active Crohn's disease? A meta-analysis of the randomized clinical trials. *JPEN J Parenter Enteral Nutr.* 1995 Sep-Oct;19(5):356-64.

Fernández-Bañares F, Cabré E, González-Huix F, Gassull MA. Enteral nutrition as primary therapy in Crohn's disease. *Gut.* 1994 Jan;35(1 Suppl):S55-9.

Fernández-Bañares F, Mingorance MD, Esteve M, et al. Serum zinc, copper, and selenium levels in inflammatory bowel disease: effect of total enteral nutrition on trace element status. *Am J Gastroenterol.* 1990 Dec;85(12):1584-9.

Fujimura Y, Honda K, Sato I, et al. Remarkable improvement of growth and developmental retardation in Crohn's disease by parenteral and enteral nutrition therapy. *Intern Med.* 1992 Jan;31(1):39-43.

Fukuda Y, Kosaka T, Okui M, Hirakawa H, Shimoyama T. Efficacy of nutritional therapy for active Crohn's disease. *J Gastroenterol.* 1995 Nov;30 Suppl 8:83-7.

Furukawa H, Yamada M, Sakurai T, Takenaka K, Matsui T, Yao T. Enteral nutrition and total parenteral nutrition in Crohn's disease; factors influencing induction of remission [in Japanese]. *Nippon Shokakibyo Gakkai Zasshi.* 1997 Dec;94(12):813-25.

Gailhoustet L, Goulet O, Cachin N, Schmitz J. Study of psychological repercussions of two modes of treatment of adolescents with Crohn's disease [in French]. *Arch Pediatr.* 2002 Feb;9(2):110-6.

Galandiuk S, O'Neill M, McDonald P, Fazio VW, Steiger E. A century of home parenteral nutrition for Crohn's disease. *Am J Surg.* 1990 Jun;159(6): 540-4; discussion 544-5.

Gassull MA, Abad A, Cabré E, González-Huix F, Giné JJ, Dolz C. Enteral nutrition in inflammatory bowel disease. *Gut.* 1986 Nov;27 Suppl 1:76-80.

Gassull MA, Fernández-Bañares F, Cabré E, et al. Fat composition may be a clue to explain the primary therapeutic effect of enteral nutrition in Crohn's disease: results of a double blind randomised multicentre European trial. *Gut.* 2002 Aug;51(2):164-8.

Gavin J, Anderson CE, Bremner AR, Beattie RM. Energy intakes of children with Crohn's disease treated with enteral nutrition as primary therapy. *J Hum Nutr Diet.* 2005 Oct;18(5):337-42.

Giaffer MH, Cann P, Holdsworth CD. Long-term effects of elemental and exclusion diets for Crohn's disease. *Aliment Pharmacol Ther.* 1991 Apr;5(2):115-25.

Giaffer MH, Holdsworth CD, Duerden BI. Effects on [sic] an elemental diet on the faecal flora in patients with Crohn's disease. *Microbial Ecol Health Dis.* 1991;4:369-74.

Giaffer MH, North G, Holdsworth CD. Controlled trial of polymeric versus elemental diet in treatment of active Crohn's disease. *Lancet.* 1990 Apr 7;335(8693):816-9.

Gineston JL, Davion T, Favi M. Cyclic enteral nutrition and Crohn's disease localized in the distal ileum and/or the colon. Trial of a dietary polymer mixture [in French]. *Ann Gastroenterol Hepatol (Paris).* 1989 Mar-Apr;25(2):41-5.

Ginsberg AL, Albert MB. Induction of remission in Crohn's disease with an Ensure diet: identification and exclusion of dietary substances which exacerbate disease [abstract]. *Gastroenterology*. 1988 May;94(5 Pt 2):A147.

Ginsberg AL, Albert MB. Treatment of patient with severe steroid-dependent Crohn's disease with nonelemental formula diet. Identification of possible etiologic dietary factor. *Dig Dis Sci*. 1989 Oct;34(10):1624-8.

Ginsberg AL, Albert MB. Treatment of Crohn's disease with a non-elemental formula diet (Ensure Plus) [abstract]. *Gastroenterology*. 1989 May; 96 (5 Pt 2):A172.

Gionchetti P, Rizzello F, Helwig U, et al. Prophylaxis of pouchitis onset with probiotic therapy: a double-blind, placebo-controlled trial. *Gastroenterology*. 2003 May;124(5):1202-9.

Giorgini GL, Stephens RV, Thayer WR Jr. The use of "medical by-pass" in the therapy of Crohn's disease: report of a case. *Am J Dig Dis*. 1973 Feb;18(2):153-7.

Godeberge P, Cosnes J, Gendre JP, Le Quintrec Y. A prospective study of liver test anomalies during continuous enteral nutrition [in French]. *Ann Gastroenterol Hepatol (Paris)*. 1989 Dec;25(7):295-8.

Goh J, O'Morain CA. Review article: nutrition and adult inflammatory bowel disease. *Aliment Pharmacol Ther*. 2003 Feb;17(3):307-20.

González-Huix F, Fernández-Bañares F, Esteve-Comas M, et al. Enteral versus parenteral nutrition as adjunct therapy in acute ulcerative colitis. *Am J Gastroenterol*. 1993 Feb;88(2):227-32.

González-Huix F, de León R, Fernández-Bañares F, et al. Polymeric enteral diets as primary treatment of active Crohn's disease: a prospective steroid controlled trial. *Gut*. 1993 Jun;34(6):778-82.

Goode A, Hawkines T, Feggetter JG, Johnston ID. Use of an elemental diet for long-term nutritional support in Crohn's disease. *Lancet*. 1976 Jan 17;1(7951):122-4.

Goodman MJ. Dietary treatment of Crohn's disease. *Lancet*. 1994 Jan 8;343(8889):112-3.

Gorard DA. Enteral nutrition in Crohn's disease: fat in the formula. *Eur J Gastroenterol Hepatol*. 2003 Feb;15(2):115-8. Erratum in: *Eur J Gastroenterol Hepatol*. 2003 Apr;15(4):459.

Gorard DA, Hunt JB, Payne-James JJ, et al. Initial response and subsequent course of Crohn's disease treated with elemental diet or prednisolone. *Gut*. 1993 Sep;34(9):1198-202.

Gorman SR, Armstrong G, Allen KR, Ellis J, Puntis JW. Scarcity in the midst of plenty: enteral tube feeding complicated by scurvy. *J Pediatr Gastroenterol Nutr.* 2002 Jul;35(1):93-5.

Göschke H, Buess H, Gyr K, et al. Elementary diet as an alternative to parenteral feeding in severe gastrointestinal diseases [in German]. *Schweiz Med Wochenschr.* 1977 Jan 15;107(2):43-9.

Gottschall, E. *Breaking the vicious cycle: intestinal health through diet.* Baltimore, ON (Canada): Kirkton Press, Ltd.; 1994.

Götze H, Ptok A. Orocaecal transit time in patients with Crohn disease. *Eur J Pediatr.* 1993 Mar;152(3):193-6.

Green CJ. Existence, causes and consequences of disease-related malnutrition in the hospital and the community, and clinical and financial benefits of nutritional intervention. *Clin Nutr.* 1999 Aug;18(Suppl 2):3-28.

Greenberg GR, Feagan BG, Martin F, et al. Oral budesonide as maintenance treatment for Crohn's disease: a placebo-controlled, dose-ranging study. Canadian Inflammatory Bowel Disease Study Group. *Gastroenterology.* 1996 Jan;110(1):45-51.

Greenberg GR, Feagan BG, Martin F, et al. Oral budesonide for active Crohn's disease. Canadian Inflammatory Bowel Disease Study Group. *N Engl J Med.* 1994 Sep 29;331(13):836-41.

Greenberg GR, Fleming CR, Jeejeebhoy KN, Rosenberg IH, Sales D, Tremaine WJ. Controlled trial of bowel rest and nutritional support in the management of Crohn's disease. *Gut.* 1988 Oct;29(10):1309-15.

Greenberg M, Heuschkel R, Davies S, et al. Enteral nutrition for indeterminate colitis. A novel approach [abstract]. *JPEN J Parenter Enteral Nutr.* 1999 May;28(5):555.

Greenstein JP, Birnbaum SM, Winitz M, Otey MC. Quantitative nutritional studies with water-soluble, chemically defined diets. I. Growth, reproduction and lactation in rats. *Arch Biochem Biophys.* 1957 Dec;72(2):396-416.

Griffiths AM. Enteral nutrition in the management of Crohn's disease. *JPEN J Parenter Enteral Nutr.* 2005 Jul-Aug;29(4 Suppl):S108-12; discussion S112-7, S184-8.

Griffiths AM. Enteral nutrition: the neglected primary therapy of active Crohn's disease. *J Pediatr Gastroenterol Nutr.* 2000 Jul;31(1):3-5.

Griffiths AM, Ohlsson A, Sherman PM, Sutherland LR. Meta-analysis of enteral nutrition as a primary treatment of active Crohn's disease. *Gastroenterology.* 1995 Apr;108(4):1056-67.

Griffiths AM, Pendley FC, Issenman RM, et al. Elemental versus polymeric enteral nutrition as primary therapy for active Crohn's disease: a multi-centre pediatric randomized controlled trial [abstract 291]. *J Pediatr Gastroenterol Nutr*. 2000;31(Suppl 2):S75-S76.

Grimaud JC, Comiti Y, Thervet L, Bremondy A, Moncada K, Salducci J. Treatment of a first attack of Crohn's disease by exclusive enteral semi-elemental nutrition. Preliminary study of 13 cases [in French]. *Gastroenterol Clin Biol*. 1990;14(8-9):680-1.

Gross V, Andus T, Caesar I, et al. Oral pH-modified release budesonide versus 6-methylprednisolone in active Crohn's disease. German/Austrian Budesonide Study Group. *Eur J Gastroenterol Hepatol*. 1996 Sep;8(9):905-9.

Gross V, Andus T, Ecker KW, et al. Low dose oral pH modified release budesonide for maintenance of steroid induced remission in Crohn's disease. The Budesonide Study Group. *Gut*. 1998 Apr;42(4):493-6.

Gugler R, Jensen JC, Schulte H, Vogel R. The course of Crohn disease and side effect profile with long-term treatment using metronidazole [in German]. *Z Gastroenterol*. 1989 Nov;27(11):676-82.

Guidry JR, Eastwood TF, Curry SC. Phenytoin absorption in volunteers receiving selected enteral feedings. *West J Med*. 1989 Jun;150(6):659-61.

Gupta P, Andrew H, Kirschner BS, Guandalini S. Is *lactobacillus* GG helpful in children with Crohn's disease? Results of a preliminary, open-label study. *J Pediatr Gastroenterol Nutr*. 2000 Oct;31(4):453-7.

Guslandi M, Mezzi G, Sorghi M, Testoni PA. *Saccharomyces boulardii* in maintenance treatment of Crohn's disease. *Dig Dis Sci*. 2000 Jul;45(7):1462-4.


Hanauer SB, Feagan BG, Lichtenstein GR, et al. Maintenance infliximab for Crohn's disease: the ACCENT I randomised trial. *Lancet*. 2002 May 4;359(9317):1541-9.

Hanauer SB, Korelitz BI, Rutgeerts P, et al. Postoperative maintenance of Crohn's disease remission with 6-mercaptopurine, mesalamine, or placebo: a 2-year trial. *Gastroenterology*. 2004 Sep;127(3):723-9.

Hanauer SB, Sandborn WJ, Rutgeerts P, et al. Human anti-tumor necrosis factor monoclonal antibody (adalimumab) in Crohn's disease: the CLASSIC-I trial. *Gastroenterology*. 2006 Feb;130(2):323-33.

Hanauer S, Sandborn WJ, Persson A, Persson T. Budesonide as maintenance treatment in Crohn's disease: a placebo-controlled trial. *Aliment Pharmacol Ther*. 2005 Feb 15;21(4):363-71.

Hannon TS, DiMeglio LA, Pfefferkorn MD, Denne SC. Acute effects of enteral nutrition on protein turnover in adolescents with Crohn disease. *Pediatr Res.* 2007 Mar;61(3):356-60.

Harms B, Bremner AR, Mulligan J, Fairhurst J, Griffiths DM, Salmon T, Beattie RM. Crohn's disease post-cardiac transplantation presenting with severe growth failure and delayed onset of puberty. *Pediatr Allergy Immunol.* 2004 Apr;15(2):186-9.

Harries AD, Danis VA, Heatley RV. Influence of nutritional status on immune functions in patients with Crohn's disease. *Gut.* 1984 May;25(5):465-72.

Harries AD, Jones LA, Danis V, et al. Controlled trial of supplemented oral nutrition in Crohn's disease. *Lancet.* 1983 Apr 23;1(8330):887-90.

Harvey RF, Heaton KW. Dietary treatment of Crohn's disease. *Lancet.* 1985 Aug 24;2(8452):453-4.

Heaton KW, Thornton JR, Emmett PM. Treatment of Crohn's disease with an unrefined-carbohydrate, fibre-rich diet. *Br Med J.* 1979 Sep 29;2(6193):764-6.

Hellers G, Cortot A, Jewell D, et al. Oral budesonide for prevention of post-surgical recurrence in Crohn's disease. The IOIBD Budesonide Study Group. *Gastroenterology.* 1999 Feb;116(2):294-300.

Herxheimer A. Elemental diets in Crohn's disease. *Lancet.* 1976 Feb 14;1 (7955):365; author reply 365.

Heuschkel R. Enteral nutrition in Crohn disease: more than just calories. *J Pediatr Gastroenterol Nutr.* 2004 Mar;38(3):239-41.

Heuschkel R. Synergy between immunosuppressive therapy and enteral nutrition in the management of childhood Crohn's disease. *JPEN J Parenter Enteral Nutr.* 2005 Jul-Aug;29(4 Suppl):S160-3; discussion S163-5, S184-8.

Heuschkel RB. Enteral nutrition in children with Crohn's disease. *J Pediatr Gastroenterol Nutr.* 2000 Nov;31(5):575.

Heuschkel RB, Menache CC, Megerian JT, Baird AE. Enteral nutrition and corticosteroids in the treatment of acute Crohn's disease in children. *J Pediatr Gastroenterol Nutr.* 2000 Jul;31(1):8-15.

Heuschkel RB, Walker-Smith JA. Enteral nutrition in inflammatory bowel disease of childhood. *JPEN J Parenter Enteral Nutr.* 1999 Sep-Oct;23(5 Suppl):S29-32.

Heymsfield SB, Smith-Andrews JL, Hersh T. Home nasoenteric feeding for malabsorption and weight loss refractory to conventional therapy. *Ann Intern Med.* 1983 Feb;98(2):168-70.

Hilsden RJ, Verhoef MJ, Best A, Pocobelli G. Complementary and alternative medicine use by Canadian patients with inflammatory bowel disease: results from a national survey. *Am J Gastroenterol.* 2003 Jul; 98(7):1563-8.

Hinojosa J, Gomollón F, García S, et al. Efficacy and safety of short-term adalimumab treatment in patients with active Crohn's disease who lost response or showed intolerance to infliximab: a prospective, open-label, multicentre trial. *Aliment Pharmacol Ther.* 2007 Feb 15;25(4):409-18.

Hinojosa J, Molés JR, Nos P, et al. Efficacy of 6-mercaptopurine in the treatment of inflammatory bowel disease [in Spanish]. *Rev Esp Enferm Dig.* 1995 Nov;87(11):775-80.

Hirakawa H, Fukuda Y, Tanida N, Hosomi M, Shimoyama T. Home elemental enteral hyperalimentation (HEEH) for the maintenance of remission in patients with Crohn's disease. *Gastroenterol Jpn.* 1993 Jun;28(3):379-84.

Hiwatashi N. Enteral nutrition for Crohn's disease in Japan. *Dis Colon Rectum.* 1997 Oct;40(10 Suppl):S48-53.

Holt PR, Katz S, Kirshoff R. Curcumin therapy in inflammatory bowel disease: a pilot study. *Dig Dis Sci.* 2005 Nov;50(11):2191-3.

Horie Y, Chiba M, Miura K, et al. Crohn's disease associated with renal amyloidosis successfully treated with an elemental diet. *J Gastroenterol.* 1997 Oct;32(5):663-7.

Hull S. Enteral versus parenteral nutrition support-rationale for increased use of enteral feeding. *Z Gastroenterol.* 1985 Aug;23 Suppl:55-63.

Hunt JB, Payne-James JJ, Palmer KR, et al. A randomised controlled trial of elemental diet and prednisolone as primary therapy in acute exacerbations of Crohn's disease. *Gastroenterology.* 1989 May;96(5 Pt 2):A224.

Hyams J, Crandall W, Kugathasan S, et al. Induction and maintenance infliximab therapy for the treatment of moderate-to-severe Crohn's disease in children. *Gastroenterology.* 2007 Mar;132(3):863-73; quiz 1165-6. Epub 2006 Dec 3.

Hyams JS, Wilson DC, Thomas A, et al. Natalizumab therapy for moderate to severe Crohn disease in adolescents. *J Pediatr Gastroenterol Nutr.* 2007 Feb;44(2):185-91.

Ikeuchi H, Kusunoki M, Yanagi H, Yamamura T, Fukuda Y, Shimoyama T. Effects of elemental diet (ED) on surgical treatment in Crohn's disease. *Hepatogastroenterology.* 2000 Mar-Apr;47(32):390-2.

Ikeuchi H, Yamamura T, Nakano H, Kosaka T, Shimoyama T, Fukuda Y. Efficacy of nutritional therapy for perforating and non-perforating Crohn's disease. *Hepatogastroenterology*. 2004 Jul-Aug;51(58):1050-2.

Imes l, Pinchbeck B, Dinwoodie A, Walker K, Thomson ABR. Effect of Ensure®, a defined-formula diet, in patients with Crohn's disease. *Digestion*. 1986;35:158-69.

Imes l, Pinchbeck B, Thomson ABR. Diet counselling improves the clinical course of patients with Crohn's disease. *Digestion*. 1988;39:7-19.

Ireton-Jones C. Case problem: medical nutrition therapy for a patient with Crohn's disease. *J Am Diet Assoc*. 2000 Apr;100(4):472-5.

Israel DM, Hassall E. Prolonged use of gastrostomy for enteral hyperalimentation in children with Crohn's disease. *Am J Gastroenterol*. 1995 Jul;90(7):1084-8.

Ito K, Hiwatashi N, Kinouchi Y, Yamazaki H, Toyata T. Improvement in abnormal intestinal permeability in active Crohn's disease by an elemental diet [abstract]. *Gastroenterology*. 1992 Apr;102(4 Pt 2):A641.

Iwata M, Nakano H, Matsuura Y, et al. Intestinal permeability in Crohn's disease and effects of elemental dietary therapy [in Japanese]. *Nippon Shokakibyo Gakkai Zasshi*. 2001 Jun;98(6):636-43.

Johnson RC, Sharma AK, Fenn NJ, Carey PD. Iatrogenic intestinal obstruction secondary to removal of a PEG. *Br J Clin Pract*. 1996 Jul-Aug;50(5):287-8.

Johnson T, Macdonald S, Hill SM, Thomas A, Murphy MS. Treatment of active Crohn's disease in children using partial enteral nutrition with liquid formula: a randomised controlled trial. *Gut*. 2006 Mar;55(3):356-61. Epub 2005 Sep 14.

Jones S, Shannon H, Srivastava E, Haboubi N. A novel approach to a patient with Crohn disease and a high stoma output: a missed opportunity? *Scand J Gastroenterol*. 2004 Apr;39(4):398-400.

Jones SC, Evans SW, Lobo AJ, Ceska M, Axon AT, Whicher JT. Serum interleukin-8 in inflammatory bowel disease. *J Gastroenterol Hepatol*. 1993 Nov-Dec;8(6):508-12.

Juteau F, Jerkovic I, Masotti V, et al. Composition and antimicrobial activity of the essential oil of *Artemisia absinthium* from Croatia and France. *Planta Med*. 2003 Feb;69(2):158-61.

Karimi O, Peña AS, van Bodegraven AA. Probiotics (VSL#3) in arthralgia in patients with ulcerative colitis and Crohn's disease: a pilot study. *Drugs Today (Barc)*. 2005 Jul;41(7):453-9.

Keller J, Panter H, Layer P. Management of the short bowel syndrome after extensive small bowel resection. *Best Pract Res Clin Gastroenterol*. 2004 Oct;18(5):977-92.

Kelts DG, Grand RJ, Shen G, Watkins JB, Werlin SL, Boehme C. Nutritional basis of growth failure in children and adolescents with Crohn's disease. *Gastroenterology*. 1979 Apr;76(4):720-7.

Khoshoo V, Reifen R, Neuman MG, Griffiths A, Pencharz PB. Effect of low- and high-fat, peptide-based diets on body composition and disease activity in adolescents with active Crohn's disease. *JPEN J Parenter Enteral Nutr*. 1996 Nov-Dec;20(6):401-5.

King TS, Woolner JT, Hunter JO. Dietary treatment of active Crohn's disease. Diet is the best treatment. *BMJ*. 1997 Jun 21;314(7097):1827-8; author reply 1828.

King TS, Woolner JT, Hunter JO. Review article: the dietary management of Crohn's disease. *Aliment Pharmacol Ther*. 1997 Feb;11(1):17-31.

Kirschner BS, Klich JR, Kalman SS, deFavaro MV, Rosenberg IH. Reversal of growth retardation in Crohn's disease with therapy emphasizing oral nutritional restitution. *Gastroenterology*. 1981 Jan;80(1):10-5.

Klaassen J, Zapata R, Mella JG, Aguayo G, Alvarado D, Espinosa O, Maíz A, Zúñiga A, Quintana C. Enteral nutrition in severe ulcerative colitis. Digestive tolerance and nutritional efficiency [in Spanish]. *Rev Med Chil*. 1998 Aug;126(8):899-904.

Klein S. Elemental versus polymeric feeding in patients with Crohn's disease— is there really a winner? *Gastroenterology*. 1990 Sep;99(3):893-4.

Klein S, Rubin DC. Enteral and parenteral nutrition. In: Feldman M, Friedman LS, Brandt LJ, eds. *Sleisenger & Fordtran's gastrointestinal and liver disease : pathophysiology, diagnosis, management*. 8th ed. Philadelphia: Saunders; 2006:287-309.

Knight C, El-Matary W, Spray C, Sandhu BK. Long-term outcome of nutritional therapy in paediatric Crohn's disease. *Clin Nutr*. 2005 Oct;24(5):775-9.

Kobayashi K, Katsumata T, Yokoyama K, Takahashi H, Igarashi M, Saigenji K. A randomized controlled study of total parenteral nutrition and enteral nutrition by elemental and polymeric diet as primary therapy in active phase of Crohn's disease [in Japanese]. *Nippon Shokakibyo Gakkai Zasshi*. 1998 Nov;95(11):1212-21.

Koga H, Iida M, Aoyagi K, Matsui T, Fujishima M. Long-term efficacy of low residue diet for the maintenance of remission in patients with Crohn's disease [in Japanese]. *Nippon Shokakibyo Gakkai Zasshi*. 1993 Nov;90(11):2882-8.

Kordali S, Cakir A, Mavi A, Kilic H, Yildirim A. Screening of chemical composition and antifungal and antioxidant activities of the essential oils from three Turkish artemisia species. *J Agric Food Chem*. 2005 Mar 9;53(5):1408-16.

Kordali S, Kotan R, Mavi A, Cakir A, Ala A, Yildirim A. Determination of the chemical composition and antioxidant activity of the essential oil of *Artemisia dracunculus* and of the antifungal and antibacterial activities of Turkish *Artemisia absinthium*, *A. dracunculus*, *Artemisia santonicum*, and *Artemisia spicigera* essential oils. *J Agric Food Chem*. 2005 Nov 30;53(24):9452-8

Korelitz BI. The role of liquid diet in the management of small bowel Crohn's disease. *Inflamm Bowel Dis*. 2000 Feb;6(1):66-7; discussion 68-9.

Korelitz BI, Adler DJ, Mendelsohn RA, Sacknoff AL. Long-term experience with 6-mercaptopurine in the treatment of Crohn's disease. *Am J Gastro-enterol*. 1993 Aug;88(8):1198-205.

Korelitz BI, Present DH. Favorable effect of 6-mercaptopurine on fistulae of Crohn's disease. *Dig Dis Sci*. 1985 Jan;30(1):58-64.

Kugathasan S, Werlin SL, Martinez A, Rivera MT, Heikenen JB, Binion DG. Prolonged duration of response to infliximab in early but not late pediatric Crohn's disease. *Am J Gastroenterol*. 2000 Nov;95(11):3189-94.

Kunz AN, Noel JM, Fairchok MP. Two cases of *Lactobacillus* bacteremia during probiotic treatment of short gut syndrome. *J Pediatr Gastroenterol Nutr*. 2004 Apr;38(4):457-8.

Kuroki F, Matsumoto T, Iida M. Selenium is depleted in Crohn's disease on enteral nutrition. *Dig Dis*. 2003;21(3):266-70.

Kusumoto I. Industrial production of L-glutamine. *J Nutr*. 2001 Sep;131(9 Suppl):2552S-2555S.

Law DK, Dudrick SJ, Abdou NI. Immunocompetence of patients with protein-calorie malnutrition. The effects of nutritional repletion. *Ann Intern Med*. 1973 Oct;79(4):545-50.

Lecomte T, Contou JF, Beaugerie L, et al. Predictive factors of response of perianal Crohn's disease to azathioprine or 6-mercaptopurine. *Dis Colon Rectum*. 2003 Nov;46(11):1469-75.

Ledeboer M, Masclee AA, Biemond I, Lamers CB. Gallbladder motility and cholecystokinin secretion during continuous enteral nutrition. *Am J Gastroenterol*. 1997 Dec;92(12):2274-9.

Leenders E, Moens E, Van Damme J. Clinical experience with space diet in pediatric surgery. *Acta Paediatr Belg*. 1974;28(3):158-64.

Leiper K, Woolner J, Mullan MM, et al. A randomised controlled trial of high versus low long chain triglyceride whole protein feed in active Crohn's disease. *Gut*. 2001 Dec;49(6):790-4.

Lémann M, Chamiot-Prieur C, Mesnard B, et al. Methotrexate for the treatment of refractory Crohn's disease. *Aliment Pharmacol Ther*. 1996 Jun;10 (3):309-14.

Lémann M, Mary JY, Duclos B, et al. Infliximab plus azathioprine for steroid-dependent Crohn's disease patients: a randomized placebo-controlled trial. *Gastroenterology*. 2006 Apr;130(4):1054-61.

Lennard-Jones JE. Sulphasalazine in asymptomatic Crohn's disease. A multicentre trial. *Gut*. 1977 Jan;18(1):69-72.

Le Quintrec Y, Cosnes J, Le Quintrec M, et al. Exclusive elemental enteral diet in cortico-resistant and cortico-dependent forms of Crohn's disease [in French]. *Gastroenterol Clin Biol*. 1987 Jun-Jul;11(6-7):477-82.

Levenstein S, Prantera C, Luzi C, D'Ubaldi A. Low residue or normal diet in Crohn's disease: a prospective controlled study in Italian patients. *Gut*. 1985 Oct;26(10):989-93.

Levine A, Milo T, Buller H, Markowitz J. Consensus and controversy in the management of pediatric Crohn disease: an international survey. *J Pediatr Gastroenterol Nutr*. 2003 Apr;36(4):464-9.

Levine A, Weizman Z, Broide E, et al. A comparison of budesonide and prednisone for the treatment of active pediatric Crohn disease. *J Pediatr Gastroenterol Nutr*. 2003 Feb;36(2):248-52.

Lewis JD, Bilker WB, Brensinger C, Deren JJ, Vaughn DJ, Strom BL. Inflammatory bowel disease is not associated with an increased risk of lymphoma. *Gastroenterology*. 2001 Nov;121(5):1080-7.

Lichtenstein GR. Approach to steroid-dependent and steroid-refractory Crohn's disease. *J Pediatr Gastroenterol Nutr*. 2001 Sep;33 Suppl 1:S27-35.

Lichtenstein GR, Yan S, Bala M, Blank M, Sands BE. Infliximab maintenance treatment reduces hospitalizations, surgeries, and procedures in fistulizing Crohn's disease. *Gastroenterology*. 2005 Apr;128(4):862-9.

Lim S, Dohil R, Meadows N, Domizio P, Sanderson IR. Treatment of orofacial and ileo-colonic Crohn's disease with total enteral nutrition. *J R Soc Med*. 1998 Sep;91(9):489-90.

Lindor KD, Fleming CR, Burnes JU, Nelson JK, Ilstrup DM. A randomized prospective trial comparing a defined formula diet, corticosteroids, and a defined formula diet plus corticosteroids in active Crohn's disease. *Mayo Clin Proc*. 1992 Apr;67(4):328-33.

Lindsay JO, Whelan K, Stagg AJ, et al. Clinical, microbiological, and immunological effects of fructo-oligosaccharide in patients with Crohn's disease. *Gut*. 2006 Mar;55(3):348-55. Epub 2005 Sep 14.

Lionetti P, Callegari ML, Ferrari S, et al. Enteral nutrition and microflora in pediatric Crohn's disease. *JPEN J Parenter Enteral Nutr*. 2005 Jul-Aug;29 (4 Suppl):S173-5; discussion S175-8, S184-8.

Lochs H. Enteral nutrition-the new maintenance therapy in Crohn's disease? *Inflamm Bowel Dis*. 2007 Dec;13(12):1581-2.

Lochs H. To feed or not to feed? Are nutritional supplements worthwhile in active Crohn's disease? *Gut*. 2006 Mar;55(3):306-7.

Lochs H, Dejong C, Hammarqvist F, et al. ESPEN Guidelines on Enteral Nutrition: Gastroenterology. *Clin Nutr*. 2006 Apr;25(2):260-74. Epub 2006 May 15.

Lochs H, Egger-Schödl M, Pötzi R, Kappel C, Schuh R. Enteral feeding—an alternative to parenteral feeding in the treatment of Crohn disease? [in German]. *Leber Magen Darm*. 1984 Mar;14(2):64-7.

Lochs H, Egger-Schödl M, Schuh R, Meryn S, Westphal G, Pötzi R. Is tube feeding with elemental diets a primary therapy of Crohn's disease? *Klin Wochenschr*. 1984 Sep 3;62(17):821-5.

Lochs H, Mayer M, Fleig WE, et al. Prophylaxis of postoperative relapse in Crohn's disease with mesalamine: European Cooperative Crohn's Disease Study VI. *Gastroenterology*. 2000 Feb;118(2):264-73.

Lochs H, Meryn S, Marosi L, Ferenci P, Hörtnagl H. Has total bowel rest a beneficial effect in the treatment of Crohn's disease? *Clin Nutr*. 1983;2: 61-4.

Lochs H, Steinhardt HJ, Klaus-Wentz B, et al. Comparison of enteral nutrition and drug treatment in active Crohn's disease. Results of the European Cooperative Crohn's Disease Study. IV. *Gastroenterology*. 1991 Oct;101(4):881-8.

Löfberg R, Rutgeerts P, Malchow H, et al. Budesonide prolongs time to relapse in ileal and ileocaecal Crohn's disease. A placebo controlled one year study. *Gut*. 1996 Jul;39(1):82-6.

Logan RF, Gillon J, Earnshaw P, Ferrington C, Ferguson A. Elemental diets in treatment of acute Crohn's disease. *Br Med J*. 1981 Jan 10;282(6258): 144-5; author reply 145.

Logan RF, Gillon J, Ferrington C, Ferguson A. Reduction of gastrointestinal protein loss by elemental diet in Crohn's disease of the small bowel. *Gut*. 1981 May;22(5):383-7.

Lomer MC, Grainger SL, Ede R, et al. Lack of efficacy of a reduced microparticle diet in a multi-centred trial of patients with active Crohn's disease.
*Eur J Gastroenterol Hepatol.* 2005 Mar;17(3):377-84.

Lomer MC, Harvey RS, Evans SM, Thompson RP, Powell JJ. Efficacy and tolera-
bility of a low microparticle diet in a double blind, randomized, pilot study
in Crohn's disease. *Eur J Gastroenterol Hepatol.* 2001 Feb;13(2):101-6.

Lomer MC, Hutchinson C, Volkert S, et al. Dietary sources of inorganic
microparticles and their intake in healthy subjects and patients with
Crohn's disease. *Br J Nutr.* 2004 Dec;92(6):947-55.

Lorenz R, Weber PC, Szimnau P, Heldwein W, Strasser T, Loeschke K.
Supplementation with n-3 fatty acids from fish oil in chronic inflammatory bowel disease—a randomized, placebo-controlled, double-blind
cross-over trial. *J Intern Med Suppl.* 1989;731:225-32.

Lorenz-Meyer H, Bauer P, Nicolay C, et al. Omega-3 fatty acids and low
carbohydrate diet for maintenance of remission in Crohn's disease. A
randomized controlled multicenter trial. Study Group Members (German
Crohn's Disease Study Group). *Scand J Gastroenterol.* 1996 Aug;31(8):778-
85.

Ludvigsson JF, Krantz M, Bodin L, Stenhammar L, Lindquist B. Elemental
versus polymeric enteral nutrition in paediatric Crohn's disease: a
multicentre randomized controlled trial. *Acta Paediatr.* 2004 Mar;93(3):
327-35.

Luna-Chadid M, Pérez Calle JL, Mendoza JL, et al. Predictors of response to
infliximab in patients with fistulizing Crohn's disease. *Rev Esp Enferm Dig.*
2004 Jun;96(6):379-81; 382-4.


MacLean CH, Mojica WA, Newberry SJ, et al. Systematic review of the effects
of n – 3 fatty acids in inflammatory bowel disease. *Am J Clin Nutr.* 2005
Sep; 82(3):611-9.

Mahadevan U, Marion JF, Present DH. Fistula response to methotrexate
in Crohn's disease: a case series. *Aliment Pharmacol Ther.* 2003 Nov
15;18(10):1003-8.

Mahajan L, Oliva L, Wyllie R, Fazio V, Steffen R, Kay M. The safety of
gastrostomy in patients with Crohn's disease. *Am J Gastroenterol.* 1997
Jun;92(6):985-8.

Mahmud N, Kamm MA, Dupas JL, et al. Olsalazine is not superior to placebo
in maintaining remission of inactive Crohn's colitis and ileocolitis:
a double blind, parallel, randomised, multicentre study. *Gut.* 2001
Oct;49(4):552-6.

Maier-Dobersberger T, Lochs H. Enteral supplementation of phosphate does not prevent hypophosphatemia during refeeding of cachectic patients. *JPEN J Parenter Enteral Nutr.* 1994 Mar-Apr;18(2):182-4.

Main AN, Morgan RJ, Hall MJ, Russell RI, Shenkin A, Fell GS. Home enteral tube feeding with a liquid diet in the long term management of inflammatory bowel disease and intestinal failure. *Scott Med J.* 1980 Oct;25(4):312-14.

Malchow H, Ewe K, Brandes JW, et al. European Cooperative Crohn's Disease Study (ECCDS): results of drug treatment. *Gastroenterology.* 1984 Feb;86(2):249-66.

Malchow H, Steinhardt HJ, Lorenz-Meyer H, et al. Feasibility and effectiveness of a defined-formula diet regimen in treating active Crohn's disease. European Cooperative Crohn's Disease Study III. *Scand J Gastroenterol.* 1990 Mar;25(3):235-44.

Malchow HA. Crohn's disease and *Escherichia coli*. A new approach in therapy to maintain remission of colonic Crohn's disease? *J Clin Gastroenterol.* 1997 Dec;25(4):653-8.

Mansfield JC, Giaffer MH, Holdsworth CD. Controlled trial of oligopeptide versus amino acid diet in treatment of active Crohn's disease. *Gut.* 1995 Jan;36(1):60-6.

Mantzaris GJ, Archavlis E, Amperiadis P, Kourtessas G, Triantafyllou G. A randomized prospective trial in active Crohn's disease comparing a polymeric diet, prednisolone, and a polymeric diet plus prednisolone [abstract]. *Gastroenterology.* 1996 Apr;110(4):A955.

Mantzaris GJ, Petraki K, Sfakianakis M, et al. Budesonide versus mesalamine for maintaining remission in patients refusing other immunomodulators for steroid-dependent Crohn's disease. *Clin Gastroenterol Hepatol.* 2003 Mar;1(2):122-8.

Markowitz J, Grancher K, Kohn N, Lesser M, Daum F. A multicenter trial of 6-mercaptopurine and prednisone in children with newly diagnosed Crohn's disease. *Gastroenterology.* 2000 Oct;119(4):895-902.

Markowitz J, Grancher K, Rosa J, Aiges H, Daum F. Growth failure in pediatric inflammatory bowel disease. *J Pediatr Gastroenterol Nutr.* 1993 May;16(4):373-80.

Markowitz J, Rosa J, Grancher K, Aiges H, Daum F. Long-term 6-mercaptopurine treatment in adolescents with Crohn's disease. *Gastroenterology.* 1990 Nov;99(5):1347-51.

Marteau P, Lémann M, Seksik P, et al. Ineffectiveness of *Lactobacillus johnsonii* LA1 for prophylaxis of postoperative recurrence in Crohn's disease: a randomised, double blind, placebo controlled GETAID trial. *Gut.* 2006 Jun;55(6):842-7. Epub 2005 Dec 23.

Martín Peña G, Valero Zanuy MA, Llorente Abarca A, Acevedo Rodríguez MT. Essential fatty acid deficiency in enteral nutrition [in Spanish]. *Nutr Hosp.* 1990 Mar-Apr;5(2):123-5.

Maté J, Castaños R, García-Samaniego J, Pajares JM. Does dietary fish oil maintain the remission of Crohn's disease (CD): a study case control [abstract]. *Gastroenterology.* 1991 May;100(5 Pt 2):A228.

Maté-Jiménez J, Hermida C, Cantero-Perona J, Moreno-Otero R. 6-mercaptopurine or methotrexate added to prednisone induces and maintains remission in steroid-dependent inflammatory bowel disease. *Eur J Gastroenterol Hepatol.* 2000 Nov;12(11):1227-33.

Matsubayashi S, Sanada M. Pregnant woman with Crohn's disease maintained on oral hyperalimentation. *Nutrition.* 1995 May-Jun;11(3):300-1.

Matsueda K. Therapeutic efficacy of elemental enteral alimentation in Crohn's disease. *J Gastroenterol.* 2000;35 Suppl 12:19.

Matsueda K, Shoda R, Takazoe M, et al. Therapeutic efficacy of cyclic home elemental enteral alimentation in Crohn's disease: Japanese cooperative Crohn's disease study. *J Gastroenterol.* 1995 Nov;30 Suppl 8:91-4.

Matsui T, Ueki M, Yamada M, Sakurai T, Yao T. Indications and options of nutritional treatment for Crohn's disease. A comparison of elemental and polymeric diets. *J Gastroenterol.* 1995 Nov;30 Suppl 8:95-7.

McCamman S, Beyer PL, Rhodes JB. A comparison of three defined formula diets in normal volunteers. *Am J Clin Nutr.* 1977 Oct; 30(10):1655-60.

McIntyre PB, Wood SR, Powell-Tuck J, Lennard-Jones JE. Nocturnal nasogastric tube feeding at home. *Postgrad Med J.* 1983 Dec;59(698):767-9.

McIntyre PB, Powell-Tuck J, Wood SR, et al. Controlled trial of bowel rest in the treatment of severe acute colitis. *Gut.* 1986 May;27(5):481-5.

McKee RF, Keenan RA. Perianal Crohn's disease—is it all bad news? *Dis Colon Rectum.* 1996 Feb;39(2):136-42.

McLeod RS, Wolff BG, Steinhart AH, et al. Prophylactic mesalamine treatment decreases postoperative recurrence of Crohn's disease. *Gastroenterology.* 1995 Aug;109(2):404-13.

Meister D, Bode J, Shand A, Ghosh S. Anti-inflammatory effects of enteral diet components on Crohn's disease-affected tissues in vitro. *Dig Liver Dis.* 2002 Jun;34(6):430-8.

Meister D, Ghosh S. Effect of fish oil enriched enteral diet on inflammatory bowel disease tissues in organ culture: differential effects on ulcerative colitis and Crohn's disease. *World J Gastroenterol*. 2005 Dec 21;11(47):7466-72.

Melmed GY, Elashoff R, Chen GC, et al. Predicting a change in diagnosis from ulcerative colitis to Crohn's disease: a nested, case-control study. *Clin Gastroenterol Hepatol*. 2007 May;5(5):602-8; quiz 525.

Melnik G. Pharmacologic aspects of enteral nutrition. In: Rombeau JL, Caldwell MD, eds. *Clinical Nutrition. Enteral and Tube Feeding*. 2nd ed. Philadelphia: W.B. Saunders Company; 1990:472-509.

Meryn S, Lochs H, Kletter K, Pötzi R, Egger-Schödl. Assessment of the value of tube feeding (TF) in Crohn's disease (CD) shown by plasma protein measurements [abstract 55]. *JPEN J Parenter Enteral Nutr*. 1982 Jul-Aug;6(4):326.

Messori A, Trallori G, D'Albasio G, Milla M, Vannozzi G, Pacini F. Defined-formula diets versus steroids in the treatment of active Crohn's disease: a meta-analysis. *Scand J Gastroenterol*. 1996 Mar;31(3):267-72.

Michener WM, Wyllie R. Management of children and adolescents with inflammatory bowel disease. *Med Clin North Am*. 1990 Jan;74(1):103-17.

Middleton SJ, Rucker JT, Kirby GA, Riordan AM, Hunter JO. Long-chain triglycerides reduce the efficacy of enteral feeds in patients with active Crohn's disease. *Clin Nutr*. 1995 Aug;14(4):229-36.

Mimura T, Rizzello F, Helwig U, et al. Once daily high dose probiotic therapy (VSL#3) for maintaining remission in recurrent or refractory pouchitis. *Gut*. 2004 Jan;53(1):108-14.

Mishkin B, Yalovsky M, Mishkin S. Increased prevalence of lactose malabsorption in Crohn's disease patients at low risk for lactose malabsorption based on ethnic origin. *Am J Gastroenterol*. 1997 July;92(7):1148-53.

Mishkin S. Controversies regarding the role of dairy products in inflammatory bowel disease. *Can J Gastroenterol*. 1994 May/Jun;8(3):205-12.

Modigliani R, Mary JY, Simon JF, et al. Clinical, biological, and endoscopic picture of attacks of Crohn's disease. Evolution on prednisolone. Groupe d'Etude Thérapeutique des Affections Inflammatoires Digestives. *Gastroenterology*. 1990 Apr;98(4):811-8.

Moran A. Bowel rest and elemental diet in Crohn's disease. *Gastroenterology*. 1993 Apr;104(4):1238-9; author reply 1239.

Morin CL, Roulet M, Roy CC, Weber A. Continuous elemental enteral alimentation in children with Crohn's disease and growth failure. *Gastroenterology*. 1980 Dec;79(6):1205-10.

Morin CL, Roulet M, Roy CC, Weber A, Lapointe N. Continuous elemental enteral alimentation in the treatment of children and adolescents with Crohn's disease. *JPEN J Parenter Enteral Nutr.* 1982 May-Jun;6(3):194-9.

Motil KJ, Grand RJ, Maletskos CJ, Young VR. The effect of disease, drug, and diet on whole body protein metabolism in adolescents with Crohn disease and growth failure. *J Pediatr.* 1982 Sep;101(3):345-51.

Motil KJ, Grand RJ, Matthews DE, Bier DM, Maletskos CJ, Young VR. Whole body leucine metabolism in adolescents with Crohn's disease and growth failure during nutritional supplementation. *Gastroenterology.* 1982 Jun;82(6):1359-68.

Munkholm Larsen P, Rasmussen D, Rønn B, Munck O, Elmgreen J, Binder V. Elemental diet: a therapeutic approach in chronic inflammatory bowel disease. *J Intern Med.* 1989 May;225(5):325-31.

Nakazawa A, Hibi T. Is fish oil (n-3 fatty acids) effective for the maintenance of remission in Crohn's disease? *J Gastroenterol.* 2000;35(2):173-5.

Navarro J, Fontaine JL, Mathé JC, et al. The treatment of Crohn's disease in the child. 12 cases [in French]. *Nouv Presse Med.* 1978 Jan 21;7(3):183-8.

Navarro J, Vargas J, Cezard JP, Charritat JL, Polonovski C. Prolonged constant rate elemental enteral nutrition in Crohn's disease. *J Pediatr Gastroenterol Nutr.* 1982;1(4):541-6.

Neidich G, Schissel K, Sharp HL. Noninvasive outpatient nutritional therapy in inflammatory bowel disease. *JPEN J Parenter Enteral Nutr.* 1985 May-Jun;9(3):350-2.

Nelson LM, Carmichael HA, Russell RI, Atherton ST. Use of an elemental diet (Vivonex) in the management of bile acid-induced diarrhoea. *Gut.* 1977 Oct;18(10):792-4.

Newby EA, Sawczenko A, Thomas AG, Wilson D. Interventions for growth failure in childhood Crohn's disease. *Cochrane Database Syst Rev.* 2005 Jul 20;(3):CD003873.

Nicholls S, Domizio P, Williams CB, et al. Cyclosporin as initial treatment for Crohn's disease. *Arch Dis Child.* 1994 Sep;71(3):243-7.

Niness KR. Inulin and oligofructose: what are they? *J Nutr.* 1999 Jul;129(7 Suppl):1402S-6S.

Nightingale J, Woodward JM; Small Bowel and Nutrition Committee of the British Society of Gastroenterology. Guidelines for management of patients with a short bowel. *Gut.* 2006 Aug;55 Suppl 4:iv1-12.

Nissler S. Ambulatory nutrition therapy from the viewpoint of a patient [in German]. *Krankenpfl J.* 1989 Jun 1;27(6):78.

Nomura M, Taruishi M, Ashida T, et al. Home enteral nutrition for the maintenance of remission in patients with Crohn's disease—including comparison between Elental and Enterued [in Japanese]. *Nippon Shokakibyo Gakkai Zasshi.* 1995 Jan;92(1):32-40.

O'Brien CJ, Giaffer MH, Cann PA, Holdsworth CD. Elemental diet in steroid-dependent and steroid-refractory Crohn's disease. *Am J Gastroenterol.* 1991 Nov;86(11):1614-8.

O'Donoghue DP, Dawson AM, Powell-Tuck J, Bown RL, Lennard-Jones JE. Double-blind withdrawal trial of azathioprine as maintenance treatment for Crohn's disease. *Lancet.* 1978 Nov 4;2(8097):955-7.

Ogata H, Hibi T. Does an elemental diet affect operation and/or recurrence rate in Crohn's disease in Japan? *J Gastroenterol.* 2003;38(10):1019-21.

O'Hagan M, Wallace SJ. Enteral formula feeds interfere with phenytoin absorption. *Brain Dev.* 1994 Mar-Apr;16(2):165-7.

Okada M, Yao T, Yamamoto T, et al. Controlled trial comparing an elemental diet with prednisolone in the treatment of active Crohn's disease. *Hepatogastroenterology.* 1990 Feb;37(1):72-80.

O'Keefe SJ, Ogden J, Rund J, Potter P. Steroids and bowel rest versus elemental diet in the treatment of patients with Crohn's disease: the effects on protein metabolism and immune function. *JPEN J Parenter Enteral Nutr.* 1989 Sep-Oct;13(5):455-60.

Olaison G, Sjödahl R, Tagesson C. Glucocorticoid treatment in ileal Crohn's disease: relief of symptoms but not of endoscopically viewed inflammation. *Gut.* 1990 Mar;31(3):325-8.

Omer B, Krebs S, Omer H, Noor TO. Steroid-sparing effect of wormwood (*Artemisia absinthium*) in Crohn's disease: a double-blind placebo-controlled study. *Phytomedicine.* 2007 Feb;14(2-3):87-95. Epub 2007 Jan 19.

O'Moráin C. Crohn's disease treated by elemental diet. *J R Soc Med.* 1982 Feb;75(2):135-6.

O'Moráin C. Elemental diets in the treatment of Crohn's disease. *Proc Nutr Soc.* 1979 Dec;38(3):403-8.

O'Moráin C, Segal AW, Levi AJ. Elemental diet as primary treatment of acute Crohn's disease: a controlled trial. *Br Med J* (Clin Res Ed). 1984 Jun 23;288(6434):1859-62.

O'Moráin C, Segal AW, Levi AJ. Elemental diets in treatment of acute Crohn's disease. *Br Med J.* 1980 Nov 1;281(6249):1173-5.

O'Moráin C, Segal AM, Levi AJ, Valman HB. Elemental diet in acute Crohn's disease. *Arch Dis Child*. 1983 Jan;58(1):44-7.

O'Moráin CA. Does nutritional therapy in inflammatory bowel disease have a primary or an adjunctive role? *Scand J Gastroenterol* Suppl. 1990;172: 29-34.

Oren R, Moshkowitz M, Odes S, et al. Methotrexate in chronic active Crohn's disease: a double-blind, randomized, Israeli multicenter trial. *Am J Gastroenterol*. 1997 Dec;92(12):2203-9.

Oriuchi T, Hiwatashi N, Kinouchi Y, et al. Clinical course and longterm prognosis of Japanese patients with Crohn's disease: predictive factors, rates of operation, and mortality. *J Gastroenterol*. 2003;38(10):942-53.

Orlando A, Colombo E, Kohn A, et al. Infliximab in the treatment of Crohn's disease: predictors of response in an Italian multicentric open study. *Dig Liver Dis*. 2005 Aug;37(8):577-83.

O'Sullivan M, O'Morain C. Nutritional therapy in inflammatory bowel disease. *Curr Treat Options Gastroenterol*. 2004 Jun;7(3):191-198.

Ouraghi A, Nieuviarts S, Mougenel JL, et al. Infliximab therapy for Crohn's disease anoperineal lesions [in French]. *Gastroenterol Clin Biol*. 2001 Nov;25(11):949-56.

Ou Tim LO, Odes HS, Duys PJ, Novis BH, Bank S, Helman CA. The use of an elemental diet in gastro-intestinal diseases. *S Afr Med J*. 1976 Oct 9;50(43):1752-6.

Palder SB, Shandling B, Bilik R, Griffiths AM, Sherman P. Perianal complications of pediatric Crohn's disease. *J Pediatr Surg*. 1991 May;26(5): 513-5.

Papadopoulou A, Rawashdeh MO, Brown GA, McNeish AS, Booth IW. Remission following an elemental diet or prednisolone in Crohn's disease. *Acta Paediatr*. 1995 Jan;84(1):79-83.

Park RH, Duncan A, Russell RI. Hypolactasia and Crohn's disease: a myth. *Am J Gastroenterol*. 1990 Jun;85(6):708-10.

Park RH, Galloway A, Danesh BJC, Russell RI. Double-blind controlled trial of elemental and polymeric diets as primary therapy in active Crohn's disease. *Eur J Gastroenterol Hepatol*. 1991;3(6):483-90.

Park R, Russell R. Diets in Crohn's disease. *Lancet*. 1990 Jun 16;335(8703): 1475-76; author reply 1476.

Payne-James JJ, Silk DBA. Use of elemental diets in the treatment Crohn's disease by gastroenterologists. *Gut*. 1990 Dec;31(12):1424.

Pearson M, Teahon K, Levi AJ, Bjarnason I. Food intolerance and Crohn's disease. *Gut*. 1993 Jun;34(6):783-7.

Perazzo FF, Carvalho JC, Carvalho JE, Rehder VL. Central properties of the essential oil and the crude ethanol extract from aerial parts of *Artemisia annua* L. *Pharmacol Res.* 2003 Nov;48(5):497-502.

Perrault J, Greseth JL, Tremaine WJ. 6-mercaptopurine therapy in selected cases of corticosteroid-dependent Crohn's disease. *Mayo Clin Proc.* 1991 May;66(5):480-4.

Phylactos AC, Fasoula IN, Arnaud-Battandier F, Walker-Smith JA, Fell JM. Effect of enteral nutrition on antioxidant enzyme systems and inflammation in paediatric Crohn's disease. *Acta Paediatr.* 2001 Aug;90(8):883-8.

Pimentel M, Chang M, Chow EJ, et al. Identification of a prodromal period in Crohn's disease but not ulcerative colitis. *Am J Gastroenterol.* 2000 Dec;95(12):3458-62.

Pincus IJ, Citron BPH, Haverback BJ. Nutritional support of gastrointestinal problems with Vivonex-100. In: Lang K, Fekl W, Berg G, eds. *Balanced Nutrition and Therapy. Bilanzierte Ernährung in der Therapie.* International Symposium in Nuremberg, April 10-12, 1970. Stuttgart: Georg Thieme Verlag; 1971: 77-80.

Polk DB, Hattner JA, Kerner JA Jr. Improved growth and disease activity after intermittent administration of a defined formula diet in children with Crohn's disease. *JPEN J Parenter Enteral Nutr.* 1992 Nov-Dec;16(6): 499-504.

Poulin E, Langevin H. Home hyperalimentation through the digestive tract [in French]. *Can J Surg.* 1982 Sep;25(5):584-9.

Prantera C, Berto E, Scribano ML, Falasco G. Use of antibiotics in the treatment of active Crohn's disease: experience with metronidazole and ciprofloxacin. *Ital J Gastroenterol Hepatol.* 1998 Dec;30(6):602-6.

Prantera C, Pallone F, Brunetti G, Cottone M, Miglioli M. Oral 5-aminosalicylic acid (Asacol) in the maintenance treatment of Crohn's disease. The Italian IBD Study Group. *Gastroenterology.* 1992 Aug;103 (2):363-8.

Prantera C, Scribano ML, Falasco G, Andreoli A, Luzi C. Ineffectiveness of probiotics in preventing recurrence after curative resection for Crohn's disease: a randomised controlled trial with *Lactobacillus GG. Gut.* 2002 Sep;51(3):405-9.

Present DH, Korelitz BI, Wisch N, Glass JL, Sachar DB, Pasternack BS. Treatment of Crohn's disease with 6-mercaptopurine. A long-term, randomized, double-blind study. *N Engl J Med.* 1980 May 1;302(18):981-7.

Present DH, Rutgeerts P, Targan S, et al. Infliximab for the treatment of fistulas in patients with Crohn's disease. *N Engl J Med.* 1999 May 6;340 (18):1398-405.

Rabast U, Heskamp R. Adjuvant therapy with elemental diet in chronic inflammatory intestinal diseases. Comparative study [in German]. *Dtsch Med Wochenschr.* 1986 Feb 21;111(8):293-7.

Rabbett H, Elbadri A, Thwaites R, et al. Quality of life in children with Crohn's disease. *J Pediatr Gastroenterol Nutr.* 1996 Dec;23(5):528-33.

Raith H, Raith B. Ambulatory artificial nutrition is definitely possible and feasible. Why? From the concerned parents' viewpoint [in German]. *Krankenpfl J.* 1989 Jun 1;27(6):76-7.

Randall HT. The history of enteral nutrition. In: Rombeau JL, Caldwell MD, eds. *Clinical Nutrition. Enteral and Tube Feeding.* 2nd ed. Philadelphia: W.B. Saunders Company; 1990:1-9.

Randell T, Murphy MS. Evaluation of elemental diet therapy as a long-term strategy for managing Crohn's disease in childhood [abstract P11]. *Arch Dis Child.* 2001;84(Suppl I):A4.

Rankin GB, Watts HD, Melnyk CS, Kelley ML Jr. National Cooperative Crohn's Disease Study: extraintestinal manifestations and perianal complications. *Gastroenterology.* 1979 Oct;77(4 Pt 2):914-20.

Rao SS, Holdsworth CD, Forrest AR. Small intestinal absorption and tolerance of enteral nutrition in acute colitis. *Br Med J (Clin Res Ed).* 1987 Sep 19;295(6600):698.

Raouf AH, Hildrey V, Daniel J, et al. Enteral feeding as sole treatment for Crohn's disease: controlled trial of whole protein v amino acid based feed and a case study of dietary challenge. *Gut.* 1991 Jun;32(6):702-7.

Rasul I, Wilson SR, MacRae H, Irwin S, Greenberg GR. Clinical and radiological responses after infliximab treatment for perianal fistulizing Crohn's disease. *Am J Gastroenterol.* 2004 Jan;99(1):82-8.

Rees RG, Keohane PP, Grimble GK, Frost PG, Attrill H, Silk DB. Elemental diet administered nasogastrically without starter regimens to patients with inflammatory bowel disease. *JPEN J Parenter Enteral Nutr.* 1986 May-Jun;10(3):258-62.

Ricour C, Duhamel JF, Nihoul-Fekete C. Use of parenteral and elementary enteral nutrition in the treatment of Crohn's disease and ulcerative colitis in children [in French]. *Arch Fr Pediatr.* 1977 Jun-Jul;34(6):505-13.

Rigaud D, Cosnes J, Le Quintrec Y, René E, Gendre JP, Mignon M. Controlled trial comparing two types of enteral nutrition in treatment of active Crohn's disease: elemental versus polymeric diet. *Gut.* 1991 Dec;32(12):1492-7.

Rijk MC, van Hogezand RA, van Lier HJ, van Tongeren JH. Sulphasalazine and prednisone compared with sulphasalazine for treating active Crohn disease. A double-blind, randomized, multicenter trial. *Ann Intern Med.* 1991 Mar 15;114(6):445-50.

Riordan AM, Hunter JO, Cowan RE, et al. Treatment of active Crohn's disease by exclusion diet: East Anglian multicentre controlled trial. *Lancet.* 1993 Nov 6;342(8880):1131-4.

Riquelme AJ, Calvo MA, Guzmán AM, et al. *Saccharomyces cerevisiae* fungemia after *Saccharomyces boulardii* treatment in immunocompromised patients. *J Clin Gastroenterol.* 2003 Jan;36(1):41-3.

Ritchie JK, Wadsworth J, Lennard-Jones JE, Rogers E. Controlled multicentre therapeutic trial of an unrefined carbohydrate, fibre rich diet in Crohn's disease. *Br Med J (Clin Res Ed).* 1987 Aug 29;295(6597):517-20.

Rocchio MA, Cha CJ, Haas KF, Randall HT. Use of chemically defined diets in the management of patients with acute inflammatory bowel disease. *Am J Surg.* 1974 Apr;127(4):469-75; discussion 475.

Rodrigues AF, Johnson T, Davies P, Murphy MS. Does polymeric formula improve adherence to liquid diet therapy in children with active Crohn's disease? *Arch Dis Child.* 2007 Sep;92(9):767-70. Epub 2007 May 2.

Rolfe VE, Fortun PJ, Hawkey CJ, Bath-Hextall F. Probiotics for maintenance of remission in Crohn's disease. *Cochrane Database Syst Rev.* 2006 Oct 18;(4):CD004826.

Romano C, Cucchiara S, Barabino A, Annese V, Sferlazzas C. Usefulness of omega-3 fatty acid supplementation in addition to mesalazine in maintaining remission in pediatric Crohn's disease: a double-blind, randomized, placebo-controlled study. *World J Gastroenterol.* 2005 Dec 7;11(45):7118-21.

Rose WC. Amino acid requirements of man. *Fed Proc.* 1949 Jun;8:546-52.

Rowe AH, Rowe A Jr, Uyeyama K. Regional enteritis; its allergic aspects. *Gastroenterology.* 1953 Apr;23(4):554-71.

Royall D, Greenberg GR, Allard JP, Baker JP, Jeejeebhoy KN. Total enteral nutrition support improves body composition of patients with active Crohn's disease. *JPEN J Parenter Enteral Nutr.* 1995 Mar-Apr;19(2):95-9.

Royall D, Jeejeebhoy KN, Baker JP, et al. Comparison of amino acid v peptide based enteral diets in active Crohn's disease: clinical and nutritional outcome. *Gut.* 1994 Jun;35(6):783-7.

Ruemmele FM, Roy CC, Levy E, Seidman EG. Nutrition as primary therapy in pediatric Crohn's disease: fact or fantasy? *J Pediatr.* 2000 Mar;136(3): 285-91.

Russell RI. Home enteral nutrition with formula diets. *Z Gastroenterol.* 1985 Aug;23 Suppl:94-7.

Russell RI, Hall MJ. Elemental diet therapy in the management of complicated Crohn's disease. *Scott Med J.* 1979 Oct;24(4):291-5.

Rutgeerts P, Diamond RH, Bala M, et al. Scheduled maintenance treatment with infliximab is superior to episodic treatment for the healing of mucosal ulceration associated with Crohn's disease. *Gastrointest Endosc.* 2006 Mar;63(3):433-42; quiz 464.

Rutgeerts P, Löfberg R, Malchow H, et al. A comparison of budesonide with prednisolone for active Crohn's disease. *N Engl J Med.* 1994 Sep 29;331(13):842-5.

Ruuska T, Savilahti E, Mäki M, Ormälä T, Visakorpi JK. Exclusive whole protein enteral diet versus prednisolone in the treatment of acute Crohn's disease in children. *J Pediatr Gastroenterol Nutr.* 1994 Aug;19(2):175-80.

Sachar DB. Patterns of post-operative recurrence in Crohn's disease. *Scand J Gastroenterol.* 1990;25(Suppl 172):35-8.

Sagher FA, Miller V. Gut peptides and elemental diet in childhood Crohn's disease. *Saudi Med J.* 2001 Nov;22(11):1035.

Sagher FA, Miller V, Ward IC. Red cell fatty acid profile and elemental diet in childhood Crohn's disease. *Saudi Med J.* 2001 Oct:22(10):931.

Saint-Raymond A, Arnaud-Battandier F, Schmitz J. Constant flow alimentation in Crohn's disease of children [in French]. *Ann Gastroenterol Hepatol (Paris).* 1988 Nov;24(6):317-21.

Saklad JJ, Graves RH, Sharp WP. Interaction of oral phenytoin with enteral feedings. *JPEN J Parenter Enteral Nutr.* 1986 May-Jun;10(3):322-3.

Sakurai T, Matsui T, Yao T, et al. Short-term efficacy of enteral nutrition in the treatment of active Crohn's disease: a randomized, controlled trial comparing nutrient formulas. *JPEN J Parenter Enteral Nutr.* 2002 Mar-Apr;26(2):98-103.

Salazopyrin in the management of Crohn's disease. The Japanese Research Committee for Crohn's disease. *Gastroenterol Jpn.* 1985 Feb;20(1):71-81.

Sandborn WJ, Colombel JF, Enns R, et al. Natalizumab induction and maintenance therapy for Crohn's disease. *N Engl J Med.* 2005 Nov 3;353 (18):1912-25.

Sandborn WJ, Feagan BG, Stoinov S, et al. Certolizumab pegol for the treatment of Crohn's disease. *N Engl J Med.* 2007 Jul 19;357(3):228-38.

Sandborn WJ, Hanauer SB, Rutgeerts P, et al. Adalimumab for maintenance treatment of Crohn's disease: results of the CLASSIC II trial. *Gut.* 2007 Sep;56(9):1232-9. Epub 2007 Feb 13.

Sandborn WJ, Löfberg R, Feagan BG, Hanauer SB, Campieri M, Greenberg GR. Budesonide for maintenance of remission in patients with Crohn's disease in medically induced remission: a predetermined pooled analysis of four randomized, double-blind, placebo-controlled trials. *Am J Gastroenterol.* 2005 Aug;100(8):1780-7.

Sandborn WJ, Rutgeerts P, Enns R, et al. Adalimumab induction therapy for Crohn disease previously treated with infliximab: a randomized trial. *Ann Intern Med.* 2007 Jun 19;146(12):829-38. Epub 2007 Apr 30.

Sanderson IR, Boulton P, Menzies I, Walker-Smith JA. Improvement of abnormal lactulose/rhamnose permeability in active Crohn's disease of the small bowel by an elemental diet. *Gut.* 1987 Sep;28(9):1073-6.

Sanderson IR, Croft NM. The anti-inflammatory effects of enteral nutrition. *JPEN J Parenter Enteral Nutr.* 2005 Jul-Aug;29(4 Suppl):S134-8; discussion S138-40, S184-8.

Sanderson IR, Udeen S, Davies PS, Savage MO, Walker-Smith JA. Remission induced by an elemental diet in small bowel Crohn's disease. *Arch Dis Child.* 1987 Feb;62(2):123-7.

Sands BE, Blank MA, Patel K, van Deventer SJ; ACCENT II Study. Long-term treatment of rectovaginal fistulas in Crohn's disease: response to infliximab in the ACCENT II Study. *Clin Gastroenterol Hepatol.* 2004 Oct;2(10):912-20.

Sarles J. Exclusive enteral nutrition in Crohn disease: elemental or not? [in French]. *Gastroenterol Clin Biol.* 1988 May;12(5):500.

Sato S, Sasaki I, Naito H, et al. Management of urinary complications in Crohn's disease. *Surg Today.* 1999;29(8):713-7.

Satran L, L'Heureux PR, Sharp H. Intestinal obstruction in Crohn's disease: medical management. *Minn Med.* 1981 Nov;64(11):661-3.

Saverymuttu S, Hodgson HJ, Chadwick VS. Controlled trial comparing prednisolone with an elemental diet plus non-absorbable antibiotics in active Crohn's disease. *Gut.* 1985 Oct;26(10):994-8.

Scheurlen M, Steinhilber D, Daiss W, Clemens M, Schmidt H, Jaschonek K. Effects of an elemental diet containing fish oil on neutrophil LTB4 synthesis and membrane lipid composition. *Prog Clin Biol Res.* 1989;301:505-9.

Schneider MU, Laudage G, Guggenmoos-Holzmann I, Riemann JF. Metronidazole in the treatment of Crohn disease. Results of a controlled randomized prospective study [in German]. *Dtsch Med Wochenschr.* 1985 Nov 8;110(45):1724-30.

Schneider MU, Strobel S, Riemann JF, Demling L. Treatment of Crohn's disease with metronidazole [in German]. *Dtsch Med Wochenschr.* 1981 Sep 4;106(36):1126-9.

Schreiber S, Khaliq-Kareemi M, Lawrance IC, et al. Maintenance therapy with certolizumab pegol for Crohn's disease. *N Engl J Med.* 2007 Jul 19;357(3):239-50.

Schulthess HK, Valli C, Escher F, Asper R, Hacki WH. Esophageal obstruction in tube feeding: a result of protein precipitation caused by antacids? [in German]. *Schweiz Med Wochenschr.* 1986 Jul 19;116(29):960-2.

Schultz M, Timmer A, Herfarth HH, Sartor RB, Vanderhoof JA, Rath HC. *Lactobacillus* GG in inducing and maintaining remission of Crohn's disease. *BMC Gastroenterol.* 2004 Mar 15;4:5.

Scott DW. Addition of potassium supplements to milk-based tube feeds. *J Hum Nutr.* 1930;34:85-90.

Scrimshaw NS, Murray EB. The acceptability of milk and milk products in populations with a high prevalence of lactose intolerance. *Am J Clin Nutr.* 1988 Oct;48(4 Suppl):1083-59.

Seidman E, Griffiths A, Jones A, Issenman R, Canadian Collaborative Pediatric Crohn's Disease Study Group. Semi-elemental (S-E) diet vs prednisone in paediatric Crohn's disease. *Gastroenterology.* 1993 Apr;104(4 Pt 2):A778.

Seidman E, Jones A, Issenman R, Griffiths A. Relapse prevention/growth enhancement in pediatric Crohn's disease: multicenter randomized controlled trial of intermittent enteral nutrition versus alternate day prednisone [abstract 9]. *J Pediatr Gastroenterol Nutr.* 1996 Oct;23(3):344.

Seidman E, Justinich C, Roy CC. Use of elemental diet therapy in paediatric inflammatory bowel disease. In: Bounous G, ed. *Uses of Elemental Diets in Clinical Situations.* Boca Raton, FL: CRC Press; 1993:243-53.

Seidman E, LeLeiko N, Ament M, et al. Nutritional issues in pediatric inflammatory bowel disease. *J Pediatr Gastroenterol Nutr.* 1991 May;12(4):424-38.

Seidman EG, Lohoues MJ, Turgeon J, Bouthillier L, Morin CL. Elemental diet versus prednisone as initial therapy in Crohn's disease: early and long term results [abstract]. *Gastroenterology.* 1991;100(5 Pt 2):A250.

Semeao EJ, Jawad AF, Stouffer NO, Zemel BS, Piccoli DA, Stallings VA. Risk factors for low bone mineral density in children and young adults with Crohn's disease. *J Pediatr.* 1999 Nov;135(5):593-600.

Sentongo TA, Semeao EJ, Piccoli DA, Stallings VA, Zemel BS. Growth, body composition, and nutritional status in children and adolescents with Crohn's disease. *J Pediatr Gastroenterol Nutr.* 2000 Jul;31(1):33-40.

Silk DB. Fibre and enteral nutrition. *Gut.* 1989 Feb;30(2):246-64.

Silk DB. Proteins, peptides and amino acids: which and when? *Nestle Nutr Workshop Ser Clin Perform Programme.* 2000;3:257-71; discussion 271-4.

Silk DBA. Enteral vs parenteral nutrition. *Clin Nutr.* 2003;22 Suppl 2:S43-8.

Silvis SE, Paragas PD Jr. Paresthesias, weakness, seizures, and hypophosphatemia in patients receiving hyperalimentation. *Gastroenterology.* 1972 Apr;62(4):513-20.

Simko V, Linscheer WG. Absorption of different elemental diets in a short-bowel syndrome lasting 15 years. *Am J Dig Dis.* 1976 May;21(6):419-25.

Singleton J. Second trial of mesalamine therapy in the treatment of active Crohn's disease. *Gastroenterology.* 1994 Aug;107(2):632-3.

Singleton JW, Hanauer SB, Gitnick GL, et al. Mesalamine capsules for the treatment of active Crohn's disease: results of a 16-week trial. Pentasa Crohn's Disease Study Group. *Gastroenterology.* 1993 May;104(5):1293-301.

Smith JAR, Stoddard CJ. Elemental diets in treatment of acute Crohn's disease. *Br Med J.* 1981 Jan 10;282(6258):144; author reply 145.

Sneed RC, Morgan WT. Interference of oral phenytoin absorption by enteral tube feedings. *Arch Phys Med Rehabil.* 1988 Sep;69(9):682-4.

Stange EF, Schmid U, Fleig WE, Ditschuneit H. Exclusion diet in Crohn disease: a controlled, randomized study [in German]. *Z Gastroenterol.* 1990 Oct;28(10):561-4.

Stehr K, Böhles H, Grosse KP. Growth retardation in Crohn's disease. Disturbed rhythm of growth hormone secretion in pediatric Crohn's disease [in German]. *Fortschr Med.* 1983 Feb 17;101(7):249-50.

Stein J, German Society for Digestive and Metabolic Diseases. Guidelines of the DGVS. Nutrition [in German]. *Z Gastroenterol.* 2003 Jan;41(1):62-8.

Steinhardt HJ, Payer E, Henn B, Ewe K, Biederlack S. Enteral nutrition in acute Crohn's disease: effect of whole vs. hydrolyzed protein on nitrogen economy and intestinal protein loss. *Gastroenterology.* 1988 May;94(5 Pt 2):A443.

Ste-Marie M. Symposium on the treatment of inflammatory bowel disease in children and adolescents. Nutritional therapy. *Can J Surg.* 1982 Sep;25(5):495-8.

Stephens RV, Bury KD, DeLuca FG, Randall HT. Use of an elemental diet in the nutritional management of catabolic disease in infants. *Am J Surg.* 1972 Apr;123(4):374-9.

Stephens RV, Randall HT. Use of concentrated, balanced, liquid elemental diet for nutritional management of catabolic states. *Ann Surg.* 1969 Oct;170(4):642-68.

Stephens RV, Thompson WR, Randall HT. The use of a fortified elemental aerospace diet in the management of nutrition following massive small bowel resection. *Surg Forum.* 1968;19:381-2.

Stober B, Nützenadel W, Ullrich F. Elemental diet in Crohn's disease [in German]. *Monatsschr Kinderheilkd.* 1983 Oct;131(10):721-4.

Stokes MA, Irving MH. How do patients with Crohn's disease fare on home parenteral nutrition? *Dis Colon Rectum.* 1988 Jun;31(6):454-8.

Stolk MF, Van Erpecum KJ, Hiemstra G, Jansen JB, Van Berge-Henegouwen GP. Gallbladder motility and cholecystokinin release during long-term enteral nutrition in patients with Crohn's disease. *Scand J Gastroenterol.* 1994 Oct;29(10):934-9.

Su C, Lichtenstein GR, Krok K, Brensinger CM, Lewis JD. A meta-analysis of the placebo rates of remission and response in clinical trials of active Crohn's disease. *Gastroenterology.* 2004 May;126(5):1257-69.

Suarez FL, Savaiano DA, Levitt MD. A comparison of symptoms after the consumption of milk or lactose-hydrolyzed milk by people with self-reported severe lactose intolerance. *N Engl J Med.* 1995 Jul 6;333(1):1-4.

Summers RW, Switz DM, Sessions JT Jr, et al. National Cooperative Crohn's Disease Study: results of drug treatment. *Gastroenterology.* 1979 Oct;77(4 Pt 2):847-69.

Sutherland LR, Martin F, Bailey RJ, et al. A randomized, placebo-controlled, double-blind trial of mesalamine in the maintenance of remission of Crohn's disease. The Canadian Mesalamine for Remission of Crohn's Disease Study Group. *Gastroenterology.* 1997 Apr;112(4):1069-77.

Takagi S, Utsunomiya K, Kuriyama S, et al. Effectiveness of an 'half elemental diet' as maintenance therapy for Crohn's disease: A randomized-controlled trial. *Aliment Pharmacol Ther.* 2006 Nov 1;24(9):1333-40.

Takazoe M, Kondoh K, Hamada T, Shimada K, Iwadare J, Matsueda K. Therapeutic efficacy of elemental enteral alimentation in Crohn's fistula. *J Gastroenterol.* 1995 Nov;30 Suppl 8:88-90.

Targan SR, Feagan BG, Fedorak RN, et al. Natalizumab for the treatment of active Crohn's disease: results of the ENCORE Trial. *Gastroenterology.* 2007 May;132(5):1672-83. Epub 2007 Mar 21.

Teahon K, Bjarnason I, Pearson M, Levi AJ. Ten years' experience with an elemental diet in the management of Crohn's disease. *Gut.* 1990 Oct;31(10):1133-7.

Teahon K, Pearson M, Levi AJ, Bjarnason I. Elemental diet in the management of Crohn's disease during pregnancy. *Gut.* 1991 Sep;32(9):1079-81.

Teahon K, Pearson M, Levi AJ, Bjarnason I. Practical aspects of enteral nutrition in the management of Crohn's disease. *JPEN J Parenter Enteral Nutr.* 1995 Sep-Oct;19(5):365-8.

Teahon K, Pearson M, Smith T, Bjarnason I. Alterations in nutritional status and disease activity during treatment of Crohn's disease with elemental diet. *Scand J Gastroenterol.* 1995 Jan;30(1):54-60.

Teahon K, Smethurst P, Pearson M, Levi AJ, Bjarnason I. The effect of elemental diet on intestinal permeability and inflammation in Crohn's disease. *Gastroenterology.* 1991 Jul;101(1):84-9.

Teahon K, Venkatesan S. Fatty acid profile of plasma lipids from patients with Crohn's disease before and after 4 weeks on elemental diet ("O 28" or "Vivonex"). *Biochem Soc Trans.* 1991;19:322S.

Teramoto F, Rokutan K, Kawakami Y, et al. Effect of 4G-beta-D-galactosyl-sucrose (lactosucrose) on fecal microflora in patients with chronic inflammatory bowel disease. *J Gastroenterol.* 1996 Feb;31(1):33-9.

Thomas AG, Holly JM, Taylor F, Miller V. Insulin like growth factor-I, insulin like growth factor binding protein-1, and insulin in childhood Crohn's disease. *Gut.* 1993 Jul;34(7):944-7.

Thomas AG, Miller V, Shenkin A, Fell GS, Taylor F. Selenium and glutathione peroxidase status in paediatric health and gastrointestinal disease. *J Pediatr Gastroenterol Nutr.* 1994 Aug;19(2):213-9.

Thomas AG, Miller V, Taylor F, Maycock P, Scrimgeour CM, Rennie MJ. Whole body protein turnover in childhood Crohn's disease. *Gut.* 1992 May;33(5):675-7.

Thomas AG, Taylor F, Miller V. Dietary intake and nutritional treatment in childhood Crohn's disease. *J Pediatr Gastroenterol Nutr.* 1993 Jul;17(1):75-81.

Thomas TS, Berto E, Scribano ML, Middleton SJ, Hunter JO. Treatment of esophageal Crohn's disease by enteral feeding via percutaneous endoscopic gastrostomy. *JPEN J Parenter Enteral Nutr.* 2000 May-Jun;24(3):176-9.

Thomsen OO, Cortot A, Jewell D, et al. A comparison of budesonide and mesalamine for active Crohn's disease. International Budesonide-Mesalamine Study Group. *N Engl J Med.* 1998 Aug 6;339(6):370-4.

Thomson AB, Wright JP, Vatn M, et al. Mesalazine (Mesasal/Claversal) 1.5 g b.d. vs. placebo in the maintenance of remission of patients with Crohn's disease. *Aliment Pharmacol Ther.* 1995 Dec;9(6):673-83.

Thompson WR, Stephens RV, Randall HT, Bowen JR. Use of the "space diet" in the management of a patient with extreme short bowel syndrome. *Am J Surg.* 1969 Apr;117(4):449-59.

Tremaine WJ, Hanauer SB, Katz S, et al. Budesonide CIR capsules (once or twice daily divided-dose) in active Crohn's disease: a randomized placebo-controlled study in the United States. *Am J Gastroenterol.* 2002 Jul;97(7):1748-54.

Triantafillidis JK, Mantzaris G, Stamataki A, Asvestis K, Malgarinos G, Gikas A. Complete remission of severe scleritis and psoriasis in a patient with active Crohn's disease using Modulen IBD as an exclusive immunomodulating diet. *J Clin Gastroenterol.* 2008 May/June;42(5): 550-555.

Tsujikawa T, Satoh J, Uda K, et al. Clinical importance of n-3 fatty acid-rich diet and nutritional education for the maintenance of remission in Crohn's disease. *J Gastroenterol.* 2000;35(2):99-104.

Tursi A, Giorgetti GM, Brandimarte G, Elisei W, Aiello F. Beclomethasone dipropionate for the treatment of mild-to-moderate Crohn's disease: an open-label, budesonide-controlled, randomized study. *Med Sci Monit.* 2006 Jun;12(6):PI29-32. Epub 2006 May 29.

Ueki M, Matsui T, Yamada M, et al. Randomized controlled trial of amino acid based diet versus oligopeptide based diet in enteral nutritional therapy of active Crohn's disease [in Japanese]. *Nippon Shokakibyo Gakkai Zasshi.* 1994 Sep;91(9):1415-25.

Ursing B, Alm T, Bárány F, et al. A comparative study of metronidazole and sulfasalazine for active Crohn's disease: the cooperative Crohn's disease study in Sweden. II. Result. *Gastroenterology.* 1982 Sep;83(3):550-62.

Vaisman N, Griffiths A, Pencharz PB. Comparison of nitrogen utilization of two elemental diets in patients with Crohn's disease. *J Pediatr Gastroenterol Nutr.* 1988 Jan-Feb;7(1):84-8.

Valli C, Schulthess HK, Asper R, Escher F, Häcki WH. Interaction of nutrients with antacids: a complication during enteral tube feeding. *Lancet.* 1986 Mar 29;1(8483):747-8.

Van Gossum A, Dewit O, Louis E, et al. Multicenter randomized-controlled clinical trial of probiotics (*Lactobacillus johnsonii*, LA1) on early endoscopic recurrence of Crohn's disease after lleo-caecal resection. *Inflamm Bowel Dis*. 2007 Feb;13(2):135-42.

Van Hees PA, Van Lier HJ, Van Elteren PH, et al. Effect of sulphasalazine in patients with active Crohn's disease: a controlled double-blind study. *Gut*. 1981 May;22(5):404-9.

Verma S, Kirkwood B, Brown S, Giaffer MH. Oral nutritional supplementation is effective in the maintenance of remission in Crohn's disease. *Dig Liver Dis*. 2000 Dec;32(9):769-74.

Verma S, Holdsworth CD, Giaffer MH. Does adjuvant nutritional support diminish steroid dependency in Crohn disease? *Scand J Gastroenterol*. 2001 Apr;36(4):383-8.

Verma S, Brown S, Kirkwood B, Giaffer MH. Polymeric versus elemental diet as primary treatment in active Crohn's disease: a randomized, double-blind trial. *Am J Gastroenterol*. 2000 Mar;95(3):735-9.

Vilien M, Dahlerup JF, Munck LK, Nørregaard P, Grønbaek K, Fallingborg J. Randomized controlled azathioprine withdrawal after more than two years treatment in Crohn's disease: increased relapse rate the following year. *Aliment Pharmacol Ther*. 2004 Jun 1;19(11):1147-52.

Voitk AJ, Echave V, Feller JH, Brown RA, Gurd FN. Experience with elemental diet in the treatment of inflammatory bowel disease. Is this primary therapy? *Arch Surg*. 1973 Aug;107(2):329-33.

von Tirpitz C, Kohn C, Steinkamp M, et al. Lactose intolerance in active Crohn's disease: clinical value of duodenal lactase analysis. *J Clin Gastroenterol*. 2002 Jan;34(1):49-53.


Waki S, Kawanami C, Kanda F, et al. Severe muscle damage induced by high carbohydrate intake from elemental diet in a patient with Crohn's disease. *J Gastroenterol*. 1998 Feb;33(1):121-4.

Walker-Smith JA. Dietary treatment of active Crohn's disease. Dietary treatment is best for children. *BMJ*. 1997 Jun 21;314(7097):1827; author reply 1828.

Walker-Smith JA. Enteral nutrition in Crohn's disease in childhood. *J Pediatr Gastroenterol Nutr*. 2001 Jan;32(1):107; author reply 107.

Walker-Smith JA. Management of growth failure in Crohn's disease. *Arch Dis Child*. 1996 Oct;75(4):351-4.

Warman JI, Korelitz BI, Fleisher MR, Janardhanam R. Cumulative experience with short- and long-term toxicity to 6-mercaptopurine in the treatment of Crohn's disease and ulcerative colitis. *J Clin Gastroenterol.* 2003 Sep;37(3):220-5.

Werlin SL. Growth failure in Crohn's disease: an approach to treatment. *JPEN J Parenter Enteral Nutr.* 1981 May-Jun;5(3):250-3.

Wilschanski M, Sherman P, Pencharz P, Davis L, Corey M, Griffiths A. Supplementary enteral nutrition maintains remission in paediatric Crohn's disease. *Gut.* 1996 Apr;38(4):543-8.

Winitz M, Adams RF, Seedman DA, Davis PN, Jayko LG, Hamilton JA. Studies in metabolic nutrition employing chemically defined diets. II. Effects on gut microflora populations. *Am J Clin Nutr.* 1970 May;23(5):546-59.

Winitz M, Graff J, Gallagher N, Narkin A, Seedman DA. Evaluation of chemical diets as nutrition for man-in-space. *Nature.* 1965 Feb 20;205(4973):741-3.

Winitz M, Seedman DA, Graff J. Studies in metabolic nutrition employing chemically defined diets. I. Extended feeding of normal human adult males. *Am J Clin Nutr.* 1970 May;23(5):525-45.

Woolfson AMJ. Elemental diets in treatment of acute Crohn's disease. *Br Med J.* 1981 Jan 10;282(6258):144; author reply 145.

Woolfson AMJ, Knapp MS, Allison SP. Elemental diets in Crohn's disease. *Lancet.* 1976 Feb 14;1(7955):365.

Woolner JT, Parker TJ, Kirby GA, Hunter JO. The development and evaluation of a diet for maintaining remission in Crohn's disease. *J Hum Nutr Diet.* 1988;11(1):1-11.

Workman EM, Alun Jones V, Wilson AJ, Hunter JO. Diet in the management of Crohn's disease. *Hum Nutr Appl Nutr.* 1984 Dec;38(6):469-73.

Wright RA, Adler EC. Peripheral parenteral nutrition is no better than enteral nutrition in acute exacerbation of Crohn's disease: a prospective trial. *J Clin Gastroenterol.* 1990 Aug;12(4):396-9.

Wright S, Sanders DS, Lobo AJ, Lennard L. Clinical significance of azathioprine active metabolite concentrations in inflammatory bowel disease. *Gut.* 2004 Aug;53(8):1123–8.

Yagi M, Tani T, Hashimoto T, et al. Four cases of selenium deficiency in postoperative long-term enteral nutrition. *Nutrition.* 1996 Jan;12(1):40-3.

Yamamoto T, Nakahigashi M, Saniabadi AR, et al. Impacts of long-term enteral nutrition on clinical and endoscopic disease activities and mucosal cytokines during remission in patients with Crohn's disease: a prospective study. *Inflamm Bowel Dis.* 2007 Dec;13(12):1493-501.

Yamamoto T, Nakahigashi M, Umegae S, Kitagawa T, Matsumoto K. Acute duodenal Crohn's disease successfully managed with low-speed elemental diet infusion via nasogastric tube: a case report. *World J Gastroenterol.* 2006 Jan 28;12(4):649-51.

Yamamoto T, Nakahigashi M, Umegae S, Kitagawa T, Matsumoto K. Impact of elemental diet on mucosal inflammation in patients with active Crohn's disease: cytokine production and endoscopic and histological findings. *Inflamm Bowel Dis.* 2005 Jun;11(6):580-8.

Yamamoto T, Nakahigashi M, Umegae S, Kitagawa T, Matsumoto K. Impact of long-term enteral nutrition on clinical and endoscopic recurrence after resection for Crohn's disease: A prospective, non-randomized, parallel, controlled study. *Aliment Pharmacol Ther.* 2007 Jan 1;25(1):67-72.

Yamazaki Y, Fukushima T, Sugita A, Takemura H, Tsuchiya S. The medical, nutritional and surgical treatment of fistulae in Crohn's disease. *Jpn J Surg.* 1990 Jul;20(4):376-83.

Younoszai MK. Growth in a teenage boy with granulomatous enteritis fed "elemental diets." *Am J Dis Child.* 1977 Feb;131(2):235-6.

Zachos M, Tondeur M, Griffiths AM. Enteral nutritional therapy for induction of remission in Crohn's disease. *Cochrane Database Syst Rev.* 2007 Jan 24;(1):CD000542.

Zoli G, Carè M, Parazza M, et al. A randomized controlled study comparing elemental diet and steroid treatment in Crohn's disease. *Aliment Pharmacol Ther.* 1997 Aug;11(4):735-40.

Zunic P, Lacotte J, Pegoix M, et al. *Saccharomyces boulardii* fungemia. Apropos of a case [in French]. *Therapie.* 1991 Nov-Dec;46(6):498-9.

# INDEX

# ACKNOWLEDGMENTS

I located much of the source material for this book at the New York Academy of Medicine. I would like to thank the staff of the Academy's library for their kind assistance in locating articles, tracking down journals, and filling endless requests for photocopies. I appreciate as well the assistance I received at Weill Cornell Medical Library, the Gustave L. and Janet W. Levy Library of the Mount Sinai School of Medicine, the National Library of Medicine, and the Medical Research Library of Brooklyn at the SUNY Downstate Medical Center. I also want to thank Dr. Fred Saibil for referring me to a patient who contributed a story to this book.

The book's handsome exterior testifies to the stellar talents of cover designer Peri Poloni-Gabriel of Knockout Design (www.knock outbooks.com) and illustrator Phil Scheuer of Phil Scheuer Illustration (http://philscheuer.com). Beverly Butterfield of Girl of the West Productions (www.girlofthewest.com) designed the interior, and its inviting layout attests to her creativity and expertise.

I am deeply grateful to the individuals who shared their own or their children's experiences with enteral nutrition, and whose stories appear in the pages of this book. I also want to express my love and gratitude to my parents and sister for their support and encouragement—and their unfailingly perceptive comments on the manuscript!

# AN INVITATION TO READERS

❖

Have you tried enteral nutrition? If so, would you be willing to share your story with others? I'd like to hear about your experiences, and possibly include them in future editions of this book. Let me know how enteral nutrition worked for you: Did you reach remission? How long did it take? Would you use it again? What were the challenges and the rewards? You can submit your story at the Web site for this book, www.ibdbook.com. Names will be changed to protect your privacy and stories may be edited to fit the available space. Thank you for helping fellow patients learn what it's like to use enteral nutrition!